THE OFFICIAL GUIDE TO
MEDICAL SCHOOL ADMISSIONS

HOW TO PREPARE FOR AND APPLY TO MEDICAL SCHOOL

2018 EDITION

Association of American Medical Colleges
Washington, D.C.

The Official Guide to Medical School Admissions
2018 Edition

AAMC Staff

MSAR® Content Specialists

Tami Levin
Director, Premed and Applicant Resources

Nicole Lee
Senior MSAR Web Content Specialist

Geoffrey Young, PhD
Senior Director, Student Affairs and Programs

Design and Editing

Jordan Campbell
Director, Creative Services

Dean Trackman
Director, Editorial Services

Rashad Muhammad
Graphic Design Specialist II

Cindy Allen
Senior Editor

Corine Sprigle
Copy Editor

Consultants

Amy Addams
Director, Competency-Based Admissions

Norma Poll
Senior Director, Diversity Policy and Programs

Lauren Siegel
Senior Communications Specialist, MCAT

Kelly K. Stazyk
Senior Writer/Editor, Careers in Medicine

Dejanira Cruz
Senior Communications Specialist, AMCAS

Irena Tartakovsky
Manager, Science Policy

Sarah Conrad
Director, Advancing Holistic Review Initiative

Lindsay Roskovensky
Senior Research and Data Analyst, Data Operations and Services

Brianna Gunter
Senior Research Analyst

Julie Gilbert
Senior Education Debt Management Specialist

To order additional copies of this publication, please contact:
Association of American Medical Colleges
AAMC Store
655 K Street, NW, Suite 100
Washington, DC 20001
Phone: 202-828-0416
email: *AAMCStore@aamc.org*
website: *aamc.org/publications*

This is a publication of the Association of American Medical Colleges. The AAMC serves and leads the academic medicine community to improve the health of all. *aamc.org*

ISBN (print): 978-1-57754-178-3

ISBN (ePub): 978-1-57754-179-0

ISBN (Kindle): 978-1-57754-180-6

Printed in the United States of America. Revised annually; new edition available in early spring.

Association of American Medical Colleges

The Association of American Medical Colleges serves and leads the academic medicine community to improve the health of all.

Founded in 1876 and based in Washington, D.C., the AAMC is a not-for-profit association dedicated to transforming health care through innovative medical education, cutting-edge patient care, and groundbreaking medical research. Our members include all 151 accredited U.S. and 17 accredited Canadian medical schools; nearly 400 major teaching hospitals and health systems, including 51 Department of Veterans Affairs medical centers; and more than 80 academic societies. Through these institutions and organizations, we serve the leaders of America's medical schools and teaching hospitals and their more than 173,000 full-time faculty members, 89,000 medical students, 129,000 resident physicians , and more than 60,000 graduate students and postdoctoral researchers in the biomedical sciences.

The AAMC's many programs and services strengthen the world's most advanced medical care by supporting the entire spectrum of education, research, and patient care activities conducted by our member institutions. The AAMC and our members are dedicated to the communities we serve and are steadfast in our desire to earn and keep the public's trust for the role we play in improving the nation's health.

The AAMC develops and administers the Medical College Admission Test® (MCAT®), operates the American Medical College Application Service® (AMCAS®), and provides detailed admission information to medical schools and undergraduate premedical advisors.

Important Notice

The information in this book is based on the most recent data provided by member medical schools at the request of the Association of American Medical Colleges (AAMC).

We edited and, in some instances, condensed the material to meet space limitations. In compiling this edition, we made every reasonable effort to ensure the accuracy and timeliness of the information, and, except where noted, the information was updated as of February 2018. All the information, however, especially figures on tuition and expenses, is subject to change and is nonbinding for the medical schools listed and the AAMC. All medical schools listed in this edition, as with other educational institutions, are subject to federal and state laws prohibiting discrimination on the basis of race, color, religion, sex, age, disability, or national origin. Such laws include Title VI of the Civil Rights Act of 1964, Title IX of the Education Amendments of 1972, Section 504 of the Rehabilitation Act of 1973, the Americans with Disabilities Act, and the Age Discrimination Act of 1975, as amended. For the most current and complete information about costs, official policies, procedures, and other matters, please contact individual schools.

In applying to U.S. or Canadian medical schools, applicants need not go through any commercial agencies. The AAMC does not endorse any organization or entity that purports to help applicants gain admission to medical school, other than undergraduate premedical advisors and medical school admissions officers.

AAMC Commitment to Diversity and Inclusion

The AAMC's mission is to serve and lead the academic medicine community to improve the health of all. As the U.S. population ages and grows more diverse and disparities in health care persist, understanding the benefits of diversity and inclusion becomes critical to addressing the health of the nation. The AAMC's commitment to diversity and inclusion in medicine and biomedical research spans more than three decades, demonstrated by ongoing leadership and engagement in activities—starting as early as high school—that promote diversity and inclusion through programs, advocacy, and research. Information about AAMC initiatives is available at *aamc.org/diversity*.

Contents

Association of American Medical Colleges   *iii*

Important Notice   *iii*

AAMC Commitment to Diversity and Inclusion   *iii*

How to Use This Guide   *1*

Chapter 1
So ... You Want to Be a Doctor   *3*
Tomorrow's Doctors, Tomorrow's Cures®   *3*
Your Medical Career Driven by Your Interests   *4*
What About the Future?   *6*
Workforce Issues   *7*
A More Collaborative Approach   *8*
Immediate Steps That Lie Ahead   *8*
A Note for Career Changes or Gap-Year Applicants   *8*

Chapter 2
Academic Preparation   *11*
Premedical Preparation   *11*
Personal Attributes   *16*
Extracurricular Activities Related to Medicine   *16*
Prehealth Advisors   *17*
Special Programs   *19*

Chapter 3
Your Medical School Years: The Education
Process   *23*
Undergraduate Medical Education: An Overview   *23*
A Word About Preclinical Versus Clinical Years   *24*
The Changing Face of Medical Education   *26*
Determining How You Want to Practice Medicine   *28*
More Medical Training: Graduate
   Medical Education   *30*
Licensure and Certification: Ready to
   Practice Independently   *32*
Continuing Medical Education: Lifelong Learning   *33*

Chapter 4
Building Toward Greater Diversity   *35*
Defining Diversity   *35*
AAMC Programs and Resources   *37*
School Programs and Resources   *39*
No Advisor? Contact the NAAHP for Help   *40*

Chapter 5
All About the MCAT® Exam   *45*
The Role of the MCAT® Exam   *45*
Eligibility   *46*
How the Exam Is Structured   *46*
What the Exam Measures   *47*
MCAT Scores   *48*
Preparing for the Exam   *49*
Test Dates, Registration, and Fees   *50*
Fee Assistance Program   *51*
Testing With Accommodations   *51*
Retaking the Exam   *51*
Score Reporting   *52*
Gap Year and Career Changers: Taking the
   MCAT Exam   *52*

Chapter 6
Choosing Your Schools   *55*
The Overall Mission of the School   *55*
Kicking Off Your Research   *56*
The Educational Program   *57*
How Do GPA and MCAT Scores Factor In?   *57*
Attending Medical School in Your Home State   *58*
International Students   *58*
Public or Private?   *58*
Additional Factors to Consider   *58*
Special Regional Opportunities   *60*

Chapter 7
Applying to Medical School   *63*
Responsibilities of the Medical School Applicant   *63*
American Medical College Application Service®   *64*
AMCAS Application Sections   *64*
The Application and Admission Cycle   *66*
Personal Statements and Letters of Evaluation   *67*
Secondary Applications   *68*
Application Fees   *68*
Criminal Background Check   *69*
Fee Assistance Program   *69*
Special Note About Deferred Entry   *70*
Gap Year and Career Changers   *70*
AAMC's Application and Acceptance Protocols for
   Applicants and Admissions Officers   *70*
AMCAS Reports Provided to Medical Schools   *73*

Chapter 8
The Admission Decision *75*
Holistic Review of Medical School Applicants *76*
Experiences *76*
Concept of "Distance Traveled" *77*
Attributes *77*
Academic Metrics *78*
Making the Evaluation *79*
The Interview Is Key *79*
A Few Last Reminders for Your Interview Day *81*

Chapter 9
Applicant and Acceptee Data *85*
A Quick Look at the 2017 Entering Class *86*
Performance on the MCAT Exam *86*
Undergraduate Grade Point Average *86*
MCAT Score *89*
Sex *89*
Age *90*
Applicant and Accepted Applicant Experiences *91*
Self-Identity *92*

Chapter 10
You Can Afford Medical School *93*
Building a Strong Financial Plan *93*
Types of Financial Aid *96*
The Financial Aid Application Process *98*
How Medical Schools Determine Eligibility
    for Financial Aid *99*
Forgiveness and Repayment Assistance Programs *99*
Federal Loans and Repayment *100*
A Final Word About Financing Your
    Medical Education *100*

Chapter 11
Baccalaureate-MD Programs *103*
Purposes of These Programs *103*
How to Find and Prepare for Baccalaureate-MD
    Programs *105*
Medical Schools Offering Combined Baccalaureate-
    MD Programs, by State, 2017–2018 *106*
Medical Schools Offering Combined Baccalaureate-
    MD Programs, by Number of Years,
    2017–2018 *109*

Chapter 12
MD-PhD Programs *113*
The Education of a Physician-Scientist *113*
The Typical Program *115*
Residency Programs After Graduation *116*
Application and Admission *116*
Financing MD-PhD Programs *117*
Gap Year and Career Changers *117*
Additional Information *117*

Chapter 13
U.S. Medical Schools *121*
Medical School Admission Requirements™ Website—
    Complete U.S. Medical School Profiles *121*
U.S. Medical Schools *121*

Chapter 14
Canadian Medical Schools *127*
Selection Criteria *127*
Canadian Medical Schools *130*

Acronyms *133*

Figures, Tables, and Worksheets

Chapter 1
So ... You Want to Be a Doctor
Figure 1.1
When did you decide to study medicine? *4*
Figure 1.2
What specialties are entering medical students considering? *5*
Figure 1.3
Projected physician shortfall range, 2016–2025 *7*
Worksheet 1.1
Important Resources and Ideas for Getting Medically Related Experiences *9*

Chapter 2
Academic Preparation
Table 2.1
MCAT and GPAs for Applicants and Matriculants to U.S. Medical Schools, by Primary Undergraduate Major, 2017–2018 *12*
Table 2.2
How Do Students Prepare for Medical School? *13*
Figure 2.1
Undergraduate major distribution, all applicants, 2012–2016 *14*
Table 2.3
Subjects Often Required or Recommended by U.S. Medical Schools *14*
Worksheet 2.1
MSAR® Premed Coursework Progress Tracker *20*
Worksheet 2.2
Journal Template for Keeping Track of Lab, Volunteer, and Work Experiences *21*

Chapter 3
Your Medical School Years: The Education Process
Figure 3.1
The most common elective and volunteer activities in medical schools, by percentage of students who participated *26*
Table 3.1
Examples of Topics in Medical Education *27*
Table 3.2
U.S. Residents by Specialty, 2016–2017 *31*

Figure 3.2
Medical school graduates' answers when asked whether they planned to become certified in a specific specialty *32*
Worksheet 3.1
Thinking About Medical Specialties *34*

Chapter 4
Building Toward Greater Diversity
Figure 4.1
Applicants to U.S. medical schools, by race, ethnicity, and sex, 2016–2017 *36*
Figure 4.2
Parental income of entering medical students, 2017 *36*
Table 4.1
Matriculants, by Medical School, Race, and Ethnicity, 2017 *41*
Worksheet 4.1
Identifying Premed and Application Programs *44*

Chapter 5
All About the MCAT® Exam
Figure 5.1
Sample MCAT score report *49*
Worksheet 5.1
Getting Ready to Take the MCAT® Exam Checklist *53*

Chapter 6
Choosing Your Schools
Figure 6.1
Matriculating students' responses to this question: In choosing the medical school you now (or will) attend, how important were the following factors? *59*
Worksheet 6.1
Factors to Weigh Before Applying *61*

Chapter 7
Applying to Medical School
Worksheet 7.1
Identifying Your Letter Writers *74*

Chapter 8
The Admission Decision
Table 8.1
Core competencies for Entering Medical Students
Endorsed by the AAMC Group on Student
Affairs Committee on Admissions   *83*
Worksheet 8.1
Possible Questions to Ask During Interviews   *84*

Chapter 9
Applicant and Acceptee Data
Figure 9.1
MCAT total score distribution, 2017 applicants   *87*
Figure 9.2
Grade point average (GPA) total distribution,
2017 applicants   *87*
Table 9.1
MCAT Total Scores and Total GPAs of Applicants
and Acceptees, 2016–2017 (Aggregated)   *88*
Figure 9.3
Applicants by sex and acceptance status,
1992–2017   *89*
Figure 9.4
Age distribution, 2017 applicants   *90*
Figure 9.5
Percentage of AMCAS applicants and accepted
applicants reporting selected experiences,
2002–2017   *91*
Figure 9.6
Distribution of self-identity,
all applicants, 2014–2017   *92*

Chapter 10
You Can Afford Medical School
Table 10.1
Tuition, Fees, and Health Insurance for 2017–2018
First-Year Students in U.S. Medical Schools
(in Dollars)   *94*
Figure 10.1
Distribution of financial aid among medical
students   *94*

Figure 10.2
Medical Student Education: Debt, Cost, and Loan
Repayment Fact Card   *96*
Table 10.2
Federal Student Loans for Medical Students   *97*
Worksheet 10.1
Monthly Budget Worksheet   *102*

Chapter 11
Baccalaureate-MD Programs
Worksheet 11.1
Baccalaureate-MD Programs to Consider
Applying To   *111*

Chapter 12
MD-PhD Programs
Worksheet 12.1
MD-PhD Programs to Consider Applying To   *119*

Chapter 14
Canadian Medical Schools
Table 14.1
Subjects Often Required or Recommended
by Canadian Medical Schools   *128*
Table 14.2
Tuition and Student Fees for 2017–2018
First-Year Students at Canadian Medical Schools
(in Canadian Dollars)   *129*
Worksheet 14.1
Questions About Canadian Medical Schools
to Ask During Interviews   *131*

**Worksheets at the end of chapters in this
guide are available in fillable PDF format
at *aamc.org/msar-resources*.**

How to Use This Guide

The AAMC works through many avenues to support medical education and help aspiring physicians succeed in their path to medical school. We created this guide to serve as a resource for students who are considering a career as a physician. Each chapter explains one aspect of the medical school admission process, and each is carefully reviewed every year by content experts at the AAMC.

Some of you may choose to read this book cover to cover, while others may prefer to skip ahead to chapters that are most relevant to where you are in the application process. Here are some tips to get the most out of the guide.

Skim the table of contents before you begin reading.
Not everyone takes the same path or is in the same place when they use this guide. You may want to read the chapters in the order that most relates to where you are now and what you need to know to move forward.

Use and update the chapter worksheets.
At the end of each chapter, you'll find a worksheet that can help you with your medical school application. Topics include keeping track of your volunteer experiences, finding individuals to write your letters of evaluation, and determining the right time to take the MCAT exam. You may want to complete some of these worksheets after you read the chapter, or you may want to hold onto them until you're at that phase of the application process. You can make copies or complete them using a fillable PDF form at *aamc.org/msar-resources*.

We encourage you to share your work with your prehealth advisor as you fill the worksheets out. You should have an advisor or a mentor to help guide you through this process. Find out more about the benefits of working with an advisor in Chapter 2, "Academic Preparation." If you do not have a prehealth advisor at your school, you can find one at *NAAHP.org*.

Look through the data in this book to understand the national picture.
Part of what will make you a well-prepared applicant will be knowing more about the national applicant and acceptance data. While every applicant is different, and while every medical school accepts applicants with a range of scores and experiences, it can be helpful to see how you compare with other applicants across the country. This will help you to decide, along with your prehealth advisor, when you're ready to apply to medical school. The data in this book come directly from the AAMC Data Warehouse, the AAMC Data Book, the American Medical College Application Service® (AMCAS®), the Medical College Admission Test® (MCAT®), and surveys conducted with entering and graduating medical students such as the Graduation Questionnaire (GQ) and the Matriculating Student Questionnaire (MSQ). The data are comprehensively updated each year with the most current information available at the time of printing. Because it comes directly from the source, you can trust that it is the most up-to-date and accurate information available. For more and current information, you can check the AAMC Facts Tables available at *aamc.org/facts*.

Check out the Medical School Admission Requirements site when you're ready to look at schools individually.
One of the most important decisions you'll make is where to apply to medical school. The AAMC's Medical School Admission Requirements™ website provides the most comprehensive, up-to-date information and data. When you're ready to start researching medical schools, tap into this powerful online database of information on U.S. and Canadian medical schools and baccalaureate-MD programs at *aamc.org/msar*. As the gold standard for admission requirement information, this is the only comprehensive resource of accurate and current data that comes directly from the MCAT program, the AMCAS program, and medical school admissions offices. Your one-year subscription allows you to search, sort, and save information.

The AAMC has resources to help you, from inspiration through practice.
We've got numerous resources to help you whether you're just beginning to consider a career as a physician or you're in the middle of applying to medical school. Take a look at these premed and applicant resources and tell other applicants about them if you find them useful.

- Aspiring Docs®

    o   Aspiring Docs Diaries (*aspiringdocsdiaries.org*)

    o   Inspiring Stories (*aamc.org/students/aspiring/inspiring-stories*)

    o   Fact Sheets (*aamc.org/students/aspiring/community/fact_sheets*)

    o   Ask a Medical Student (*youtube.com/user/AAMCvideo*)

- Financial Aid and Financial Literacy Resources

    o   Fact Sheets (*aamc.org/first/factsheets*)

    o   MedLoans® Organizer and Calculator (*aamc.org/services/first/medloans*)

    o   SALT: Money knowledge for college—and beyond (*saltmoney.org/AAMC*)

- Medical College Application Test® (MCAT®)

    o   *MCAT® Essentials* (*students-residents.aamc.org/mcatessentials*)

    o   Official Guide to the MCAT® Exam (*aamc.org/students/applying/mcat/mcat2015*)

- American Medical College Application Service® (AMCAS®)

    o   *2018 AMCAS® Applicant Guide* (*aamc.org/amcasguide*)

- Careers in Medicine® (CiM) (*aamc.org/cim*)

Keep up and communicate with us on social media.
One of the best ways to find out about what's going on is to follow us on Facebook and Twitter and to check out our videos on YouTube:

   Facebook: *facebook.com/aamcpremed*

Twitter: *twitter.com/aamcpremed*

   YouTube: *youtube.com/user/AAMCvideo*

A note about "MD versus DO" programs: This guidebook explains the process of preparing for and applying to medical doctor (MD) programs accredited by the Liaison Committee on Medical Education (LCME). You may have heard of osteopathic medicine programs that grant doctor of osteopathic medicine (DO) degrees. DO and MD programs have many similarities; both types of physicians are fully certified to practice medicine in the United States after passing board examinations. For more information about DO-granting schools and admission requirements, consult the American Association of Colleges of Osteopathic Medicine site (*aacom.org*).

CHAPTER 1

So ... You Want to Be a Doctor

First, I want to congratulate you on your decision to explore medical school and a career in medicine. This is the first step into a remarkable and wonderful field.

When I decided medicine was my path, I talked to my mother, who is a nurse. She shared how challenging life as a doctor is—the difficult training, the long hours, the high expectations. She emphasized that being a doctor is not as glamorous as television makes it seem. I am grateful for her insight because it forced me to evaluate the reasons behind my decision. I looked at my shadowing and volunteering experiences differently and discovered a love of medicine and patient care that drove me to work even harder to achieve my goal of becoming a doctor. These experiences helped me to realize there is nothing else that I could imagine myself doing even with the tremendous effort required and the consistent difficulties along the path.

Now in my third year of medical school, I can say this love of interacting with patients and using my passion for science and medicine to improve lives is what has kept me going through the challenges. It is what gets me through a long day in the hospital or the stress of studying for an exam, and it is the same motivation that energized me when I was in your position applying to medical school.

I encourage you to dig deep and find your core motivation. Let this motivation guide your application, and it will be what carries you through the challenges ahead. This guidebook will help you through the nitty-gritty of the application process, but never lose sight of the reason why being a doctor is what you are meant to do.

Nicholas Beam
MD Candidate
Western Michigan University
Homer Stryker MD School of Medicine
Class of 2018

Tomorrow's Doctors, Tomorrow's Cures®

The dream of becoming a doctor is something that many applicants seem to know from an early age. In fact, a recent AAMC survey shows that half of all medical students who responded to the survey had chosen a medical career before they set foot in college—and one in five had made the choice before they even started high school (see Figure 1.1).

Whether you have always known that you wanted to be a doctor or are just starting to consider the idea, being a physician is an extremely rewarding profession. A career in medicine offers numerous opportunities to make a real difference in the lives of countless people.

As a doctor, you are likely to see new life come into the world or provide comfort to those about to leave it. Or you may choose to help build the future of medicine by educating the next generation of physicians. Perhaps you will dedicate yourself to discovering new cures for devastating diseases.

Whichever direction you follow, you will play a role in reducing or eliminating people's pain and suffering, improve their quality of life, and provide invaluable service to your local community or the country as a whole.

Figure 1.1. When did you decide to study medicine? Most applicants knew early on that they wanted to be a doctor.

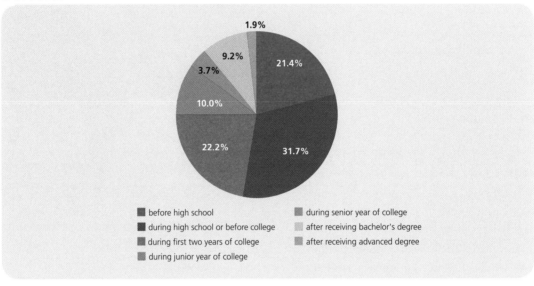

Source: AAMC's 2017 Matriculating Student Questionnaire (MSQ).

Your Medical Career Driven by Your Interests

Another benefit of the field is that you can choose from many and varied ways to practice. From clinical practice to biomedical research, from public health to medical education—the choices are plentiful (see Figure 1.2). Medical students typically have clear preferences for the areas they plan to specialize in after graduation. Many students change or further refine their specialty preferences as they gain experience and knowledge in medical school. If your interests change with time and experience, medicine—because of its emphasis on lifelong learning and ties to research and technological developments—will provide you with opportunities to refine your skills and reorient your practice. Here are some examples of possible career options:

- The satisfaction of long-term patient relationships is one attraction of **family medicine and internal medicine**, where the bulk of time is spent in direct contact with patients. Physicians who work under the umbrella of "primary care" often care for entire families and enjoy the challenges that come from treating a diverse population with varied backgrounds and conditions.

- Other physicians may prefer to pursue detailed knowledge about the intricacies of a single organ or system, such as that required of **cardiologists, ophthalmologists, dermatologists, endocrinologists,** and other specialists.

- Interested in **scientific exploration** and the desire to **break new ground in medical knowledge**? Physicians with these interests are found in the nation's private and public laboratories and research institutions.

- Those with a commitment to social justice and an interest in fulfilling the health care needs of the underserved and disadvantaged can meet those challenges **in urban and rural clinics, in public health, or as medical missionaries**.

- Careers in **general surgery** often suit people who have a desire to see immediate results of their interventions. **Plastic and reconstructive surgery** draws others with artistic skills and aesthetic interests.

- Those interested in mind-body interactions and the emotional lives of their patients might find a home in **neurology or psychiatry.**

- The fast pace of medicine draws some to work as **emergency physicians or trauma surgeons**.

- Others motivated by the interest of national defense may use their skills as **flight surgeons or in military medicine**.

- The **economic and public policy aspects of health care** guide some physicians to think tanks and health-related organizations, as well as to serve in the legislative and executive branches of government.

- For those fascinated by the issues facing groups of patients with age-defined illnesses and problems— from the risks in infancy and early childhood to the challenges of older life—fulfillment can come in careers as **pediatricians and geriatricians**.

- Assisting patients in overcoming complex fertility and gestational problems is the hallmark of the specialists in **reproductive endocrinology and obstetrics and gynecology**.

- Those dedicated to reducing the incidence of birth defects and inherited diseases might find their calling in **medical genetics**.

- The detection, prevention, and eradication of injury and disease draw people to the fields of **preventive medicine and epidemiology**.

Once you enter medical school, you'll start actively learning about these and the myriad other career options and considering where you best fit. This is addressed further in Chapter 3, in the section "Determining How You Want to Practice Medicine."

Figure 1.2. What specialties are entering medical students considering?

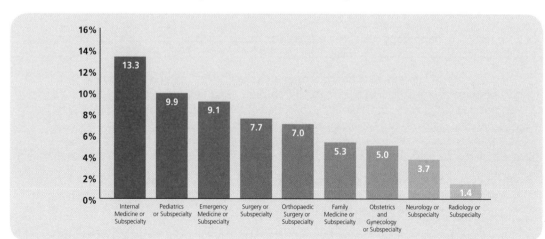

Source: AAMC's 2017 Matriculating Student Questionnaire (MSQ).

What About the Future?

As long as we're looking ahead, let's look way ahead. In 5, 10, 15 years, what will medicine look like?

One thing is certain—the face of medicine changes continually. A good example of this has to do with the prevalence of women in medicine. In the 1976–1977 academic year, women made up just 24.7% of all medical school matriculants. Compare that with 2017–2018, when they made up half— 50.7%—of the entering class, according to the AAMC Applicant Matriculant File.

Medical students taking the Hippocratic Oath, 2015.

Look back one generation, and you can see that many new fields have emerged.

- An excellent example dates back to the early 1980s. Back then, a new—and fatal—illness was taking hold that nobody could identify. We now know it well: AIDS. **Infectious disease** is currently a large medical subspecialty, and, as a result, significant advances have been made in extending the lives of those infected with HIV.

- Other advances are more recent. In last few decades, **minimally invasive surgery**, in which surgeons carry out precise procedures sometimes with the assistance of a robot, became increasingly popular. Such surgeries are currently available and used in procedures on lungs, the esophagus, the prostate, the uterus, and kidneys. Through surgeries like these, patients are likely to benefit from smaller incisions, lower risk of complications, shorter hospital stays, less pain, and speedier recoveries.

- **Personalized medicine**, a career path unavailable to the previous generation, is a field where the technology allows physicians to identify mutated genes and alert patients about their predisposition to a specific disease. (The next step—actually treating diseases with genes—is on the horizon.)

- Then, there are the more established fields that have evolved to take on new applications. Radiology, for example, is no longer about just reading X-rays. Radiologists can now perform surgery as part of **interventional radiology**.

Even more exciting is what lies ahead: gene therapy, portable medical records, distance surgery, and focused medication. The possibilities for advancement in medical research are limitless.

- Early tests of **gene therapy** have been especially favorable for cystic fibrosis, in which the correct CFTR gene is transported via a harmless virus or liposome.

- Similarly, research is under way in **pharmacogenomics**, a field that uses patients' genetic codes to develop tailored treatments. For example, if a patient's genes fit a certain type of cancer code, the physician will prescribe the "matching" pharmaceutical that has been developed to destroy cells with that code and will know, rather than hope, that the treatment is likely to work. Pharmacogenomics is still in its infancy, with most forms of tailored drugs used in oncology, but studies are progressing in other areas, including cardiology, diabetes, and psychiatric disorders.

- Also in development is **focused preventive care**, which uses genetic diagnosis to identify to a very specific degree how likely a patient is to develop a certain disease or condition—and then prevents that development before it has a chance to begin.

- Other advances will be administrative in nature; the days of hunting down medical records may come to an end, for example. One possibility being explored is a **portable medical records** system, or a national online database of individual health records. Everyone will carry a smart card (or have an implanted microchip!), allowing physicians easy access to medical records. The benefit? Errors are reduced, files are readily available, delays are minimized or eliminated, and the experience of having repeated—that is, unnecessary—tests is eliminated.

Workforce Issues

Above all, know this: Whatever specialty you choose, your services as a physician will be needed.

According to a study commissioned by the AAMC, there will be a shortage of 61,700 to 94,700 physicians by 2025. The shortage is being driven in large part by the rapid expansion of the number of Americans age 65 or over. Our doctors are getting older, too. Nearly one-third of today's physicians will be of retirement age in the next decade, just as more Americans need care. A continued demand for physicians and other medical professionals is projected.

Figure 1.3 illustrates the growing physician shortages between 2016 and 2025. Still, the shortages will be experienced unevenly, and some geographic areas will feel the effect more strongly than others. With that in mind, you might consider the trends as you think about the direction you'd like your career to take.

Figure 1.3. Projected physician shortfall range, 2016–2025.

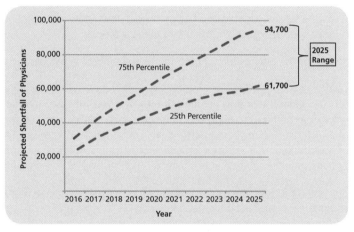

Source: AAMC Center for Workforce Studies, 2016 (aamc.org/2016projections).

Primary Care

Although the nation is facing an overall shortage of physicians, many people are particularly concerned about the growing deficit of primary care doctors. Within the overall shortage of physicians, experts expect a shortfall of between 14,900 and 35,600 primary care physicians by 2025. To encourage U.S. medical school graduates to pursue a career in primary care, the federal government and many state governments offer a variety of scholarship and loan repayment programs. You may want to explore the rewards this type of career offers, including the satisfaction that comes from delivering comprehensive care and having long-term relationships with your patients.

Underserved Areas

The impact of this shortage is expected to be greatest in underserved areas—the urban and rural areas where health care is already scarce. If you choose to serve in a community designated as a Health Professional Shortage Area by the U.S. Department of Health and Human Services, you may be able to take advantage of a federal program—the National Health Service Corps—that offers scholarships and loan repayment. According to the AAMC's 2017 Matriculating Student Questionnaire, about 29% of entering students planned to work in a primarily underserved area, and more than half of entering student survey participants hadn't yet decided where they wanted to work. (Learn more about this program in Chapter 10, "You Can Afford Medical School.")

A More Collaborative Approach

As Congress explores various scenarios as it moves forward with instituting health care reform, one thing is nearly certain: Given the projected shortage of physicians, we will need to develop new models of health care delivery that make better, more efficient use of all health care professionals—not just doctors. That means you can expect to work within a more collaborative, "shared" environment, in which a team of health care providers—physician's assistants and nurse practitioners, for example—work more in tandem. Exactly how that will play out is still in development, but the goal is to create a more efficient system, increase patient satisfaction, and, ultimately, improve health outcomes.

A collaborative approach to health care delivery is instilled beginning in the early years of medical education. Read more about the use of small-group discussions, problem-based learning, and other educational models in Chapter 3, "Your Medical School Years: The Education Process."

Immediate Steps That Lie Ahead

That's the future—or at least what we expect. Right now, though, you're undoubtedly more focused on the short-term goal of getting into medical school.

So what *is* the process for applying to medical school? What lies ahead?

Let's be candid. Getting into medical school isn't easy. (But it's definitely doable—as the more than 89,904 students currently enrolled can testify!) You will need to prepare for and take the MCAT® exam, select schools to apply to, complete the application, write a personal statement, gather letters of evaluation, secure your undergraduate transcripts, and interview. And then you will wait for notices of acceptance and make your final decision. If you're not accepted, you'll need to evaluate your options and figure out what to do next. All of this will be covered in the following chapters.

But first, right now, you can take many steps to make yourself a more attractive candidate to admission committees. From taking the necessary courses to working effectively with your prehealth advisor to participating in extracurricular and volunteer activities, there's a lot you can do.

In the next chapter, we focus on your undergraduate preparation.

A Note for Career Changers or Gap-Year Applicants

If a year or more has passed since you graduated from college, you're not alone. Well over half (62.6%) of matriculating medical students indicated in the AAMC's Matriculating Student Questionnaire that there was a gap between their college graduation and matriculation to medical school of at least a year. Medical schools do not see a break between the end of college and beginning of medical school as a weakness or negative attribute. In fact, what you've experienced or accomplished during this time may enhance your application and qualifications significantly.

We'll add tips and things to consider throughout this book to help guide you through the application and preparation process. We know there may be some variation in how you'll need to prepare yourself and compile the different components of your application now that you're no longer on campus.

 Worksheets at the end of chapters in this guide are available in fillable PDF format at *aamc.org/msar-resources*.

Advising Office

Your prehealth advisor*:_____

Advising office phone number: _____

Advisor's email address: _____

Office location: _____

*If your school does not have prehealth advising or you don't have access to an advisor, see the National Association of Advisors for the Health Professions' (NAAHP's) Find an Advisor service (*naahp.org/StudentResources/FindanAdvisor.aspx*).

Clubs and Volunteer Opportunities

Premed club or society on campus: _____

Premed honor society:_____

Service organization club or fraternity: _____

Other Ideas to Make Contacts and Get Experience:

❏ Contact science department about lab and/or research opportunities.

Notes: _____

_____

_____

❏ Contact local clinic or health service provider for volunteer, paid, part-time, or internship opportunities.

Notes: _____

_____

_____

❏ Contact health care providers you know about shadowing opportunities.

Notes: _____

_____

_____

_____

CHAPTER 2

Academic Preparation

> *Sometimes as a second-year medical student, I think about how far I've come since high school, when I was volunteering at my local hospital. It was just 15 minutes from home, but it opened my eyes to medicine. From that moment, I was hooked! I said yes to every shadowing opportunity and searched for more. I once asked my mentor if I could shadow overnight at the hospital. You honestly could not get me to leave!*
>
> *As a premed, every moment of shadowing is a new experience. It is as thrilling and exciting for me as the first time I felt it. In addition to shadowing, while in college, I reached out to professors I'd had classes with to see if they had research opportunities I could get involved in. While these inquiries only finally panned out in senior year, they were incredibly rewarding, gave me great letters of recommendation, and got me interested in research! I also volunteered to TA two of my favorite science classes—a not-so-novel way to give back, which actually helped with my understanding of the course material. And from freshmen year until graduation, I served on the Student Volunteer Emergency Medical Service, getting to experience my earliest patient encounters.*
>
> *Ultimately, the journey of a premed, and really any aspiring doctor, is one of enterprise and endurance. A doctor once said, "It's the people who have the most stamina who ultimately end up on top," and truer words were never spoken.*

Ogochukwu Marietta Ezeoke
MD Candidate
State University of New York
Upstate Medical University
Class of 2019

Premedical Preparation

College coursework plays a major role in your preparation for medical school. Your major field of study, the mastery of specific scientific principles, and advanced coursework all contribute to that preparation. Let's take a closer look at each of these.

Choice of Major

Contrary to what many college students believe, there is no such thing as the "best" major. **In fact, no medical school requires a specific major of its applicants**. That's because admissions committee members know that students develop the essential skills of acquiring and synthesizing information through a wide variety of academic disciplines and, therefore, should be free to select whichever major they find interesting and challenging.

Even so, many premedical students choose to major in a scientific discipline. If that's the direction you're heading in, and you're doing so because you are fascinated by science and believe that such a major will be the foundation for a variety of career options, great. If you're doing so because you believe it will enhance your chances for admission, think again.

Admissions committees welcome students whose intellectual curiosity leads them to a wide variety of disciplines.

The table below displays MCAT scores and GPAs for applicants and matriculants to U.S. medical schools for 2017–2018 by primary undergraduate major. MCAT scores and GPAs are displayed by mean or median and standard deviation (SD). Please email *datarequest@aamc.org* if you have questions about the table.

Table 2.1. MCAT and GPAs for Applicants and Matriculants to U.S. Medical Schools, by Primary Undergraduate Major, 2017–2018

Applicants	MCAT CPBS Mean	SD	MCAT CARS Mean	SD	MCAT BBLS Mean	SD	MCAT PSBB Mean	SD	Total MCAT Mean	SD	GPA Science Mean	SD	GPA Non-Science Mean	SD	GPA Total Mean	SD	Total Applicants
Biological Sciences	126.1	2.8	125.5	2.7	126.5	2.7	126.4	2.7	504.5	9.3	3.46	0.42	3.72	0.28	3.56	0.34	28,204
Humanities	126.5	2.7	126.9	2.6	126.7	2.7	127.2	2.6	507.4	8.8	3.42	0.46	3.70	0.28	3.57	0.32	1,776
Math and Statistics	127.7	2.5	126.7	2.8	127.2	2.6	127.3	2.6	508.9	8.8	3.54	0.39	3.70	0.30	3.59	0.34	336
Other	125.9	2.8	125.6	2.7	126.1	2.8	126.4	2.8	504.0	9.4	3.45	0.43	3.69	0.29	3.56	0.34	9,585
Physical Sciences	127.2	2.7	126.0	2.7	126.7	2.7	126.7	2.7	506.7	9.3	3.52	0.40	3.67	0.31	3.58	0.33	4,787
Social Sciences	125.9	2.8	126.1	2.7	126.0	2.8	127.0	2.7	505.0	9.2	3.37	0.46	3.63	0.32	3.51	0.34	5,333
Specialized Health Sciences	125.2	2.8	125.0	2.8	125.4	2.8	125.8	2.9	501.3	9.8	3.39	0.47	3.67	0.31	3.53	0.35	1,659
All Applicants	*126.2*	*2.8*	*125.7*	*2.7*	*126.4*	*2.8*	*126.5*	*2.8*	*504.7*	*9.4*	*3.45*	*0.43*	*3.70*	*0.29*	*3.56*	*0.34*	*51,680*

Matriculants	MCAT CPBS Mean	SD	MCAT CARS Mean	SD	MCAT BBLS Mean	SD	MCAT PSBB Mean	SD	Total MCAT Mean	SD	GPA Science Mean	SD	GPA Non-Science Mean	SD	GPA Total Mean	SD	Total Matriculants
Biological Sciences	127.6	2.2	126.7	2.3	127.9	2.1	127.9	2.1	510.1	6.7	3.65	0.30	3.81	0.21	3.71	0.25	11,534
Humanities	127.7	2.2	127.8	2.2	128.0	2.1	128.3	2.1	511.8	6.6	3.61	0.32	3.78	0.21	3.70	0.23	888
Math and Statistics	128.7	1.9	127.4	2.4	128.2	1.9	128.3	2.2	512.6	6.2	3.70	0.29	3.78	0.23	3.73	0.25	162
Other	127.5	2.1	126.9	2.3	127.7	2.1	128.0	2.1	510.2	6.4	3.63	0.31	3.78	0.22	3.71	0.24	3,789
Physical Sciences	128.4	2.1	127.1	2.4	128.0	2.1	127.9	2.1	511.5	6.7	3.69	0.27	3.77	0.24	3.72	0.24	2,182
Social Sciences	127.4	2.2	127.3	2.2	127.6	2.2	128.5	2.0	510.8	6.4	3.58	0.33	3.73	0.26	3.66	0.26	2,204
Specialized Health Sciences	127.0	2.2	126.6	2.3	127.3	2.0	127.8	2.1	508.7	6.4	3.61	0.33	3.79	0.22	3.70	0.25	579
All Matriculants	*127.6*	*2.2*	*126.9*	*2.3*	*127.9*	*2.1*	*128.0*	*2.1*	*510.4*	*6.6*	*3.64*	*0.31*	*3.79*	*0.22*	*3.71*	*0.25*	*21,338*

Note: In April 2015, the AAMC launched a new version of the MCAT exam. Scores are reported in four sections: 1) Chemical and Physical Foundations of Biological Systems (CPBS), 2) Critical Analysis and Reasoning Skills (CARS), 3) Biological and Biochemical Foundations of Living Systems (BBLS), and 4) Psychological, Social, and Biological Foundations of Behavior (PSBB). Because of this change, the 2016 and 2017 MCAT scores are not comparable to previous years, and 2017 scores are not comparable to 2016 scores. In 2017, 11.5% of the applicants applied with scores from the old version of the MCAT® exam only, 15.9% applied with scores from the old exam and the new exam, and 71.0% applied with scores from the new exam only. The MCAT columns include data from 44,869 applicants and 18,074 matriculants in 2017. The GPA columns include data from 51,432 applicants and 21,165 matriculants in 2017.

And no … you won't be at a disadvantage if you choose to major in English, for example, rather than biology. You may be surprised to learn that there is very little difference in median total MCAT® scores among those who major in the humanities, social sciences, and biological sciences. Table 2.1 shows that students from many different majors are accepted to medical school, as long as they have the basic science preparation.

College students take advantage of a variety of programs to prepare for medical school and a career in medicine. Table 2.2 shows the percentage of students who participated in several popular programs.

Scientific Preparation

Still, medical schools recognize the importance of a strong foundation in mathematics and the natural sciences—biology, chemistry, and physics—and most schools have established minimum course requirements for admission. These courses usually represent about one-third of the credit hours needed for degree completion (leaving room for applicants to pursue a broad spectrum of college majors, as shown in Figure 2.1). Many medical schools have progressed to competency-based admissions, meaning they do not require specific courses. For those that do require courses, they typically expect that their entering students will have mastered basic scientific principles by successfully completing one academic year (two semesters or three quarters) each of biology, physics, general chemistry, and organic chemistry, including adequate laboratory experiences. Increasingly, biochemistry is strongly recommended by schools, too.

Table 2.2. How Do Students Prepare for Medical School?

Program	Proportion of Students
Health care field volunteer	92.5%
MCAT® preparation course	57.1%
Laboratory research apprenticeship	59.6%
Summer academic enrichment	14.7%
Nondegree postbaccalaureate program to complete premedical requirements	8.9%
Nondegree postbaccalaureate program to strengthen academic skills	7.1%

Source: AAMC's 2017 Matriculating Student Questionnaire (MSQ). https://www. aamc.org/download/485324/data/msq2017report.pdf

Figure 2.1 presents information about the undergraduate majors of all medical school applicants to entering classes for the years 2012–2016. Over the past five years, more than half of all applicants reported undergraduate biological science majors, while the remainder reported a variety of majors, including the humanities, mathematics and statistics, physical sciences, social sciences, and other health sciences, and a broad "other" category. The proportion of these majors has remained relatively constant over time, despite annual fluctuations in the numbers of applicants.

Although only a few medical schools require applicants to complete a specific course in mathematics, all schools appreciate that mathematical competence provides a strong foundation for understanding basic sciences. A working knowledge of statistics helps students fully grasp medical literature. Many medical schools therefore recommend coursework in mathematics and statistics in addition to the science courses named above. Table 2.3 gives an overview of the most common courses required or recommended by medical schools.

AP, IB, and CLEP Courses

If you intend to apply college credit earned through **advanced placement (AP), international baccalaureate (IB), and college-level examination placement (CLEP)** to meet premedical requirements, you should be aware that some medical schools have requirements involving the use of such credit. Please review the Medical School Admission Requirements™ (MSAR®) website (*aamc.org/msar*) and the websites of medical schools you're interested in for more information.

Figure 2.1. Undergraduate major distribution, all applicants, 2012–2016.

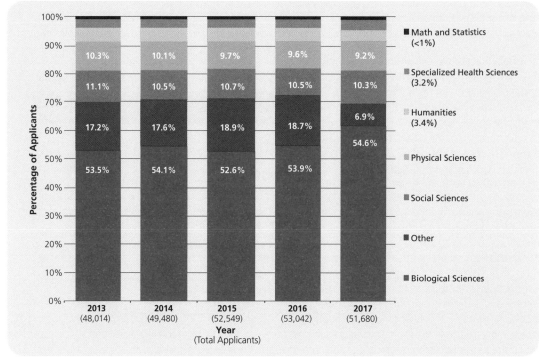

Source: AAMC Data Warehouse: Applicant Matriculant File.

Competencies Versus Courses

Finally, for those of you reading this in the early years of college (or in high school), we would like to draw your attention to the fact that medical schools are increasingly defining their prerequisites by competencies—rather than courses. This comes about because, as a collaborative report between the Howard Hughes Medical Institute (HHMI) and the AAMC points out, the scientific knowledge medical schools seek in their applicants can be obtained in a variety of courses as opposed to specific ones. In other words, a student might be able to develop and apply knowledge about chemistry principles in a zoology class or statistics in a sociology class. (The AAMC-HHMI report *The Scientific Foundations for Future Physicians* is available at *aamc.org/scientificfoundations*.)

Advanced Coursework

Although upper-level science coursework may not be required by every medical school, it's usually a good idea to show that you have challenged yourself academically. Successfully completing advanced courses demonstrates science proficiencies and ultimately strengthens your preparation for medical school. Taking science courses that simply duplicate basic content, however, is not recommended. But don't think that all your

Table 2.3. Subjects Often Required or Recommended by U.S. Medical Schools*

Required or Recommended Subject
Biochemistry
Biology
Biology/Zoology
Calculus
College Mathematics
English
Humanities
Inorganic Chemistry
Organic Chemistry
Physics
Social Sciences

*For specific requirements and recommendations, see the individual school profiles on the Medical School Admission Requirements™ website: aamc.org/msar (subscription required). You can also view coursework requirements on individual medical school websites. Source: AAMC Medical School Admission Requirements website, 2016.

upper-level courses must be STEM-based (science, technology, engineering, and math). Practicing physicians often suggest that premedical students take advantage of what might be their final opportunity for formal study in nonscience areas and take elective courses in subjects of interest, such as music, art, history, and literature. Medical schools are also looking for applicants with rich and varied coursework and experiences. Beyond that, medical schools encourage honors courses, independent study, and research work by premedical students. Activities such as these demonstrate in-depth scholarly exploration and the presence of the lifelong-learning skills that are essential to a career in medicine.

Career Changers and Gap-Year Students: Not All Coursework Is "Evergreen"

It's important for applicants who have had a significant break between completing coursework and applying to medical school to check with the schools or look at the MSAR site for details on the oldest date coursework can be accepted. This is especially important for core premedical requirements, though some schools may waive the requirement for individual courses based on an applicant's professional experience (for instance, an applicant whose current work shows a high level of competency in a medically related area). Be sure to contact the schools you're interested in or check their websites for their requirements, or look at the MSAR site.

Some applicants who may need to complete numerous courses choose to do so via postbaccalaureate premedical programs for career changers or for those who need to enhance their academic record. Postbaccalaureate information is available on the AAMC's free postbaccalaureate database (*apps.aamc.org/postbac/#/index*).

Competencies for Entering Medical Students

The AAMC's Core Competencies for Entering Medical Students were developed to highlight the knowledge, skills, values, and attributes that the medical education community thinks are fundamental for students and future physicians. The competencies fall into three categories: Preprofessional, Thinking and Reasoning, and Science (*aamc.org/admissions/dataandresearch/477182/corecompetencies.html*). One of the most essential core competencies is **Cultural Competence**, which states that applicants should:

- Demonstrate knowledge of sociocultural factors that affect interactions and behaviors

- Show appreciation and respect for multiple dimensions of diversity

- Recognize and act on the obligation to inform one's own judgment

- Engage diverse and competing perspectives as a resource for learning, citizenship, and work

- Recognize and appropriately address bias in themselves and others

- Interact effectively with people from diverse backgrounds

The *Scientific Foundations for Future Physicians* AAMC-HHMI report proposes scientific competencies for future medical school graduates and undergraduate students who want to pursue a career in medicine, including these:

- Both the knowledge of and ability to apply basic principles of mathematics and statistics, physics, chemistry, biochemistry, and biology to human health and disease

- The ability to demonstrate observational and analytical skills

- The ability to apply those skills and principles to biological situations

These scientific competencies have been incorporated into the AAMC's Thinking and Reasoning and Science Core Competencies.

Personal Attributes

As the Core Competencies for Entering Medical Students suggest, academic and scientific accomplishments alone are not sufficient preparation for medical school. While intellectual capacity is obviously important to being a successful physician, so are other attributes that signify the ability to develop and maintain effective relationships with patients, work collaboratively with other team members, act ethically and compassionately, and in many other ways master the "art" of medicine.

The AAMC publication *Learning Objectives for Medical Student Education: Guidelines for Medical Schools* describes the personal attributes required of a physician (*aamc.org/initiatives/msop*). While making note of the fact that graduating medical students must be knowledgeable about medicine and skillful in its application, the publication also emphasizes how vital it is for students to:

- Make ethical decisions

- Act with compassion, respect, honesty, and integrity

- Work collaboratively with team members

- Advocate on behalf of one's patients

- Be sensitive to potential conflicts of interest

- Be able to recognize one's own limits

- Be dedicated to continuously improving one's knowledge and abilities

- Appreciate the complex nonbiological determinants of poor health

- Be aware of community and public health issues

- Be able to identify risk factors for disease

- Be committed to early identification and treatment of diseases

- Accept responsibility for making scientifically based medical decisions

- Be willing to advocate for the care of the underserved

Chances are, some of the most valuable traits you'll demonstrate as a physician are not going to be learned in a classroom. These characteristics may be nurtured throughout your college years (and, as you will see in Chapter 8, are among the attributes that admissions officers seek when admitting applicants to their programs). You don't need formal programs to learn how to be a kind, empathetic physician. You'll have an abundance of opportunities to develop these qualities through your interactions with friends, classmates, and others while in college and through your life, work, and volunteer experiences.

Extracurricular Activities Related to Medicine

Your undergraduate years offer opportunities to become involved in a wide range of extracurricular activities. Ideally, at least a few of them should involve the medical field. Experience in a health care setting, such as volunteering at shelters or clinics or in other environments to care for ill or elderly people in your community; participating in basic or clinical research efforts; working as an emergency medical technician; "shadowing" a physician; and providing support to people in a rape crisis center, emergency room, or social service agency are all types of activities recommended to those considering a career in medicine.

These pursuits give you the chance to learn more about the medical profession and yourself. You will, for example, be able to:

- Explore different interests

- Be able to experience and evaluate different working environments

- Better understand the nature of medical practice and the daily demands placed on physicians

- Assess your ability to communicate and empathize with people from different backgrounds and cultures

- Evaluate your willingness to put others' needs before your own

While this self-analysis can help you decide if a career in medicine is right for you, your involvement with clinical or research activities also helps demonstrate to admissions committees where your interests lie. It shows that you have explored various aspects of the medical field.

Admissions committees evaluate your experiences using at least three different criteria, and a greater value is assigned to some types of pursuits than others. Specifically, admissions committees look at the length of time you've invested, the depth of the experience, and lessons learned—in relation to any particular activity. This means a single, daylong blood drive or one-time-only shadowing experience is often perceived as less enlightening than semester or yearlong commitments. By the same token, active participation in an activity is viewed as more instructive than passive participation (such as observation). Most important, admissions committees want to know what students learned from their experiences. You should be prepared to address questions about your community, clinical, or research experiences in your application materials (which will be discussed in Chapter 7, "Applying to Medical School").

Do *not* approach your extracurricular activities with the idea of "checking off" a wide range of pursuits to impress admissions committees. Three or four in-depth experiences from which you gained valuable lessons are far more significant—and telling—to admissions officers than dozens of short-term involvements.

Prehealth Advisors

Fortunately, you're not on your own when it comes to preparing for medical school. Valuable resources are available to you—some of which are likely to be right on campus, including your prehealth advisor.

Depending on the individual school, prehealth advisors work on a full- or part-time basis and may be a faculty member (often in a science department), a staff member in the office of an academic dean or in the career center, the director or staff in an advising office for preprofessional students, or a physician in part-time practice. Advisors belong to organizations such as the National Association of Advisors for the Health Professions (NAAHP, *naahp.org*) that assist them in their work—and help them help you. If your school does not have a prehealth advisor, contact the NAAHP about getting a member volunteer to help you. Visit *naahp.org/StudentResources/FindanAdvisor.aspx* for more information. You can find a link to each school's admission requirements page here, *students-residents.aamc.org/choosing-medical-career/article/required-premedical-coursework-and-competencies*, and you can use the Medical School Admission Requirements website to view each school's admission requirement profile. You can always reach out to medical school admissions staff if you have specific questions about admission requirements or policies. Be sure to check the medical school's website first, though, to see if the information is available there.

Services Provided

The support provided by prehealth advisors varies from school to school. Be sure to contact your school's advisor to find out which services and resources are offered.

Generally speaking, services fall into five categories:

- **Academics.** Advisors are well-informed about premedical coursework on their campuses and often work with faculty at their schools to develop suitable academic programs for premed students. They collaborate with campus academic staff to design study, reading skills, and test-preparation workshops; offer tutoring programs; and inform students they advise about regional and national programs likely to be of interest.

- **Clinical and research experiences.** Advisors often work with advisory groups composed of college and medical school teaching and research faculty and community clinicians. They help applicants identify part-time jobs, volunteer positions, and opportunities for independent study credit in local laboratories and offices.

- **Advising and support.** Advisors help students pursue realistic goals and maximize their potential, both meeting with them individually and providing group opportunities for students to meet with one another. Advisors often establish peer advising and mentoring programs and are particularly sensitive to the needs of students who are underrepresented in medicine or are the first in their family to attend college.

- **Assistance to student organizations.** Advisors coordinate the activities of local and national organizations that serve premed students by planning programs, identifying funding sources, and arranging for campus visits from admissions and financial aid officers.

- **Sharing resources.** Advisors disseminate publications and other resources from relevant organizations, including the AAMC and NAAHP, to meet students' need for timely and pertinent information. In addition, advisors provide access to web-based content on health careers programs and educational financing; distribute information about local, regional, national, and international research and service opportunities; and stock a library of publications related to medical school and medical education.

A Wide Range of Guidance

A prehealth advisor may assist you in many ways, including:

- Identifying courses that satisfy premedical requirements

- Determining a sequence for completing those courses

- Finding tutorial assistance, if needed

- Planning academic schedules to accommodate both premed coursework and other educational objectives, such as a study program abroad, a dual major, or a senior honors thesis

- Locating volunteer or paid clinical and research experience

- Strengthening your medical school application

- Preparing for interviews and standardized tests

- Arranging for letters of evaluation

- Determining the most appropriate career paths based on your strengths, values, and life goals

Letters of Evaluation and Committee Letters

There is another vital service that many prehealth advisors offer their students (and often their alumni): the prehealth committee letter of evaluation.

This is usually a composite letter written on behalf of a medical school applicant by the college or university's prehealth committee. It presents an overview of the student's academic strengths, exposure to health care and medical research environments, contributions to the campus and community, and personal attributes such as maturity and altruism. In addition, the letter may address any extenuating circumstances that may have resulted in deficits in the student's performance during a course or semester, provide perspective on challenges the student may have encountered, and explain school-specific courses and programs in which the student has participated.

Some undergraduate institutions do not provide composite letters of evaluation but instead collect individual letters throughout the student's enrollment. Then, at the appropriate time, they distribute the letters to the medical schools where the student has applied. Keep in mind that letter of evaluation distribution, practices, and polices vary at each undergraduate institution. Under the Admissions section of the MSAR site, you can find more information about each school's letter policy. It's a good idea to work with your prehealth advising office to clarify how they intend to send letters on your behalf.

Special Programs

Finally, we would like to draw your attention to the following two programs that may be of interest (depending on where you fall in the education process).

Combined Baccalaureate-MD Programs

If you're reading this book during the last year or two of high school, you might want to explore a combined baccalaureate-MD program, offered at about a quarter of U.S. medical schools. Graduates of these programs, which range in length from six to nine years, receive both a bachelor's degree from the undergraduate institution and an MD from the medical school. For more details and a list of participating schools, please see Chapter 11 (*aamc.org/msar*).

Postbaccalaureate Programs

Perhaps you're at a different stage along the educational continuum and have already graduated from college. If your major was something other than science, it's possible that you may need to pursue additional coursework before applying to medical school. Postbaccalaureate programs offered at colleges and universities across the country range from formal one- or two-year master's degree programs to certificate programs. They are available to help applicants who may need to strengthen their knowledge in the sciences, complete required premedical coursework, or enhance their academic background or who are career changers. A searchable database of these programs can be found at *apps.aamc.org/postbac/#/index*. You can also locate medical schools that have postbaccalaureate programs using the search features on the Medical School Admission Requirements website (*aamc.org/msar*).

 Worksheets at the end of chapters in this guide are available in fillable PDF format at *aamc.org/msar-resources*.

Use this worksheet to keep track of your completed premedical courses. The Medical School Admission Requirements™ (MSAR) website includes charts of each medical school's premedical coursework requirements (*aamc.org/msar*). To compare your completed coursework with all medical schools' requirements, use the My Coursework feature available to MSAR subscribers.

Course	Completed	Enrolled	Needed	N/A*	Notes
Behavioral Sciences					
Biochemistry					
Biology					
Biology/Zoology					
Calculus					
College English					
College Mathematics					
Computer Science					
Genetics					
Humanities					
Inorganic Chemistry					
Organic Chemistry					
Physics					
Psychology					
Social Sciences					

*N/A = not applicable because it's not required.

Journal Template for Keeping Track of Lab, Volunteer, and Work Experiences

This worksheet will come in handy when you're writing application essays, tracking your experiences, identifying people to ask for letters of evaluation, and filling out the American Medical College Application Service® (AMCAS®) application. You can fill out the online form at *aamc.org/msar-resources*.

Date	Experience	What I did	How this prepares or influences me	# of hours	Contact name email, and phone
[Example] January 15– April 1, 2018	Shadowing	Observed Dr. Addams in primary care role	I was able to observe patient-physician interactions and learned about an electronic medical record system.	25	

CHAPTER 3

Your Medical School Years: The Education Process

You think you'll be ready. You walk into a patient's room, white coat sharply creased, stethoscope neatly tucked into your pocket. You think back on how many times you practiced, the checklists you memorized, the lecture slides you pored over—and you think surely you're prepared. Until the moment you walk in. Your heart races, pounding so hard that when you press down to take the patient's pulse, the only one you can feel is your own.

Because to stand, even if only for a moment, as the authority figure at the foot of the bed, to shoulder, even if only briefly, the hopes and fears of another human—nothing really prepares you for that.

But of course, this is why you are here. It's terrifying at first. Slowly you realize the hours you spent on neuropathology have allowed you to read a radiology report on a head CT and understand it. When patients list their medications, the names are becoming familiar. The attending asks if you could hear the heart murmur. Tentatively, you answer yes, and then realize this time, you are sure.

Day by day, the new becomes familiar—the foreign, comprehensible. You start to see, you start to hear, you start to know. And you realize there will come a day—not today, not tomorrow, but someday—when it will be you who writes the report, who selects the prescriptions, who diagnoses the murmur. A day when you can do this.

Nihaal Mehta
MD Candidate
Warren Alpert Medical School
of Brown University
Class of 2019

Undergraduate Medical Education: An Overview

At the core, all U.S. medical schools have the same purpose—to educate their students in the art and science of medicine, provide them with clinical experience, and, ultimately, prepare them to enter the next phase of medical training. That is why every school follows the same basic program, requiring students to acquire a basic foundation in the medical sciences, apply this knowledge to diseases and treatments, and master clinical skills through a series of clinical rotations. (Read more about Canadian medical schools in Chapter 14.)

That doesn't mean that all medical schools are alike. It's often said, "When you've seen one medical school, you've seen one medical school." Each institution establishes its own curriculum and course requirements, so, for example, a particular class required by one institution is an elective course in another. Even when medical schools seem to offer identical courses, the content within them may differ, so some of the material covered in immunology in one school, for instance, is presented in pathology in another. The sequence in which courses are taken—and the method by which the content is taught—may differ as well. Beyond that, the processes by which students are graded also vary from school to school, with some institutions following a pass/fail system, others an honors/pass/fail system, and still others a letter grading system. And just as the culture, campus, and personality of the undergraduate schools you considered differed, they also differ among medical schools. The process you'll use to decide which medical school is the best fit for you and your needs will likely be similar to the one you used to choose your college.

Medical schools must meet very exacting standards to earn (and maintain) accreditation, as established by the Liaison Committee on Medical Education (LCME). The LCME, cosponsored by the AAMC and the American Medical Association, accredits medical school programs that grant the MD degree in the United States (*lcme.org*). (Accreditation by the LCME is required for schools to receive federal grants and to participate in federal loan programs. In addition, eligibility of U.S. students to take the United States Medical Licensing Examination [USMLE]—a discussion of which appears on page 32—requires LCME accreditation of their school. All medical schools listed in this guide are accredited by the LCME.)

Beyond accreditation requirements, the general educational structure and curriculum of most medical schools are similar. There is significant overlap between what has traditionally been referred to as the "preclinical" and "clinical" years—commonly, the first two and last two years of medical school, respectively.

A Word About Preclinical Versus Clinical Years

Students typically concentrate their efforts on the scientific underpinnings of medicine during the first two years and apply and refine that knowledge during a series of rotations during the last two years. However, there is often an overlap in content between these two stages of medical education. It's increasingly common for a student to have some clinical exposure in the first year of medical school. Similarly, during the clinical years, students refine their understanding of underlying medical concepts and apply basic science knowledge. It's important, therefore, to recognize that preclinical and clinical content can—and does—intersect at any stage in the medical school experience.

Building a Foundation of Knowledge

In almost all cases, you'll begin your medical school studies by learning how the human body is supposed to work—in terms of both structure and function. The focus will then shift to abnormal conditions and diseases, methods of diagnosis, and treatment options.

Normal Structure and Function
Before you learn about illnesses and ailments, you'll learn how the healthy body works. That's what you'll be studying right out of the starting gate, and your courses will be many—and varied. Typically, your basic classes will include gross and microscopic anatomy, physiology, biochemistry, behavioral sciences, and neurology.

Abnormalities, Diagnostics, and Treatment
After you've learned what "healthy" looks like (and acts like), the focus of your coursework will shift again, in structure and function. You'll study the full range of diseases and atypical conditions, methods by which diagnoses are made, and therapeutic principles and treatments. It's at this stage that you'll have classes in immunology, pathology, and pharmacology.

Other Topics

You'll be exposed to a wide variety of other topics, such as nutrition, medical ethics, genetics, laboratory medicine, substance abuse, geriatrics, health care delivery systems, research, preventive medicine, human sexuality, and community health, to name a few. The subjects taught at medical schools are as varied, and potentially as numerous, as the institutions themselves.

And that's just part of the picture. There's much more to "building a foundation" than mastering the scientific basis of medicine. During this period of your medical education, you'll learn the basics of taking a patient history, conducting physical exams, interpreting laboratory findings, and considering diagnostic treatment and alternatives—in effect, readying yourself for the clinical rotations that follow in the second half of medical school.

Finally, keep in mind that practicing medicine is not all science—or even the application of science (such as that required to interpret lab results and figure out a course of treatment). Medical schools recognize that physicians practice in a social environment—one in which effective team building, collaboration, and communication skills are necessary. As a result, the very way students learn and are taught has evolved in recent years. (This is discussed in more depth on page 26 under "The Changing Face of Medical Education.")

What a Typical Curriculum May Include

Although the specifics of curricula may differ from school to school, most of them follow the same basic structure. (The list below doesn't include all possible courses and clerkships.)

Year 1: Normal structure and function—Biochemistry, cell biology, medical genetics, gross anatomy, structure and function of human organs, behavioral science, and neuroscience

Year 2: Abnormal structure and function—Abnormalities of structure and function, disease, microbiology, immunology, pathology, and pharmacology

Years 3 and 4: Clinical clerkships—Generalist core: family medicine, internal medicine, obstetrics and gynecology, pediatrics, and surgery

Other requirements: neurology, psychiatry, anesthesiology, dermatology, urology, radiology, and electives

Acquiring Hands-On Experience Through Rotations

A major component of your undergraduate medical education, typically during the third and fourth years, will be a series of clinical rotations that usually last from four to six weeks each. Under direct supervision of a faculty member, you'll get firsthand experience working with patients and their families in inpatient and outpatient settings.

What You'll Do

During a rotation, you'll be assigned to an outpatient clinic or inpatient hospital unit where you'll assume responsibility for "working up" a number of patients each week—collecting relevant data and information from them and presenting findings to a faculty member. Beyond that, you'll participate in the ongoing care of patients, either during hospitalizations or through the course of outpatient treatment. When appropriate, you'll interact not only with the patients themselves, but also with their families.

And What You'll Learn

There's no substitute for hands-on experience—and plenty of it. During the course of your rotations, you'll learn to apply basic science knowledge and clinical skills in diagnosing and treating patients' illnesses and injuries and will become adept at interacting with patients (and their families) as you provide information, answer questions, and prepare your patients for the likely outcome. At the same time, you'll become effective at working with all members of the health care team, whether at the bedside, during inpatient team discussions ("rounds"), or in case-based lectures and small-group discussions.

Electives

Just like college, you'll get an opportunity to explore special interests by way of electives. Offered in basic, behavioral, and clinical sciences, as well as in basic and clinical research, electives are usually available during your final year of medical school (although you might be able to take them at other times). They may be completed on your own campus, at other medical schools through a "visiting student program," through federal and state agencies, in international settings, and through service organizations. The range of activities medical students participate in is broad. The most popular ones are shown in Figure 3.1.

Figure 3.1. The most common elective and volunteer activities in medical schools, by percentage of students who participated.

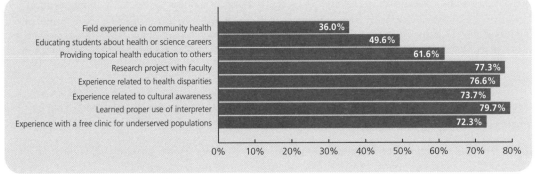

Source: AAMC's 2017 Graduation Questionnaire (GQ).

The AAMC **Visiting Student Learning Opportunities**™ (VSLO™) program is designed for medical and public health students to pursue short-term learning opportunities in locations away from their home institutions. The VSLO program merged two existing visiting student programs: the Visiting Student Application Service (VSAS®) program that focused exclusively on U.S. domestic away electives and the Global Health Learning Opportunities (GHLO®) program that facilitated international mobility into the United States, from the United States to electives abroad, and from one non-U.S. location to another. VSLO streamlines the application process for both students and institutions. Visit the VSLO website for more information: *students-residents.aamc.org/attending-medical-school/article/visiting-student-learning-opportunities/*.

The Changing Face of Medical Education

You may have heard of Abraham Flexner, who wrote a groundbreaking report on medical education in 1910, when many medical schools were small trade schools unaffiliated with a university and a degree was awarded after only two years of study. Although the basics of his model have survived to the present day—mainly, a four-year program affiliated with a university—he never intended it to serve for more than a generation. After all, no one can predict the future.

Time has certainly proven that this is a successful model.

There's no way that Flexner could have anticipated the shifting demographics, technological advances, and evolving teaching techniques of the late 20th and early 21st centuries. According to the U.S. Bureau of the Census, the U.S. population over age 65 is expected to be almost 74 million by 2030—accounting for 1 in every 5 Americans. Demographics such as that, together with advanced technologies, scientific discoveries, and evolving teaching techniques, all contribute to significant changes in medical education. You'll experience firsthand the reforms taking place in medical education, in terms of both what you'll learn and how you'll learn it. Your courses may range from cultural competency to health care financing, and you'll benefit from educational developments such as computer-aided instruction, virtual patients, and human patient simulation.

What You'll Learn

You're going to wield a scalpel in anatomy class early on in medical school, just as students in our parents' and grandparents' generations did 30 and 60 years ago. Certain things stay the same. That type of effort aside, though, there are many significant changes in medical education content, and schools are continually revising their curricula to reflect advances in science, breakthroughs in medicine, and changes in society. For example:

- Consider the demographic shift we'll experience as the baby boomers age. Physicians will spend an increasing amount of time treating age-related problems such as Alzheimer's disease, heart failure, pulmonary disease, and bone disorders. As a result, most medical schools now include in their curricula courses on geriatrics, palliative care, pain management, complementary medicine, and other similar age-based material.

- Issues such as health literacy, nutrition, drug abuse, and domestic violence are now important components of medical education. Because many of these and other health problems are related to culture and lifestyle, medical schools have increasingly focused efforts on areas such as disease prevention, health promotion, population health, and cultural diversity.

- Medical schools are focusing increasingly on helping their students develop more effective communication skills, allowing them to interact successfully with a diverse group of patients. You'll be taught specifically how to assess family, lifestyle, and socioeconomic factors that may influence your patients' behavior or affect their care.

Then, of course, there are the advances in science and medicine themselves. As researchers make breakthroughs in genetic diagnoses and treatments, for instance, that new knowledge is incorporated into the medical school program. There are also expanded courses on medical ethics, examining some of the dilemmas physicians may face amid the advent of new technology; classes on financial decision making, in which students are taught to weigh the likely costs and benefits of various treatments; and sessions on evidence-based medicine and patient quality, providing students with the information and tools they will need to deliver the best possible care. Some examples of topics that are now included in medical education are shown in Table 3.1.

The topics described here are only an overview of some possibilities. The specific courses you'll take as a medical student will vary depending on the school.

How You'll Learn It

Do you have an image of sitting in a large lecture hall, surrounded by hundreds of your peers? While you may experience that aspect of medical school, that method of teaching is being replaced (to a significant degree) by other techniques. Here are a few of the most widespread methods:

- The traditional lecture-based approach is increasingly giving way to student-

Table 3.1. Examples of Topics in Medical Education

Specialty	Number of Medical Schools Requiring the Topic*
Medical genetics	140
Cultural competence	140
Communication skills	141
Domestic violence/abuse	141
Pain management	140
Substance abuse	139
Prevention/health maintenance	139
Health care systems	139
Complementary/alternative health care	130
Medical economics	132

*n=142.
Source: 2015–2016 LCME Annual Medical School Questionnaire Part II.

centered, small-group instruction—similar to the case study teaching method common in both law and business schools. You may be assigned to small groups of students—overseen by a faculty member—in which you'll focus on specific clinical problems. The aim here is to instill medical knowledge and skills, as well as help you build the communication and collaboration skills you'll need as you continue your medical training and, ultimately, as a fully licensed physician.

- Fast-moving technological advances have certainly affected the medical school education program. You'll probably use a computerized patient simulator to apply the basic sciences you've mastered to a clinical context and refine your diagnostic skills. These simulators, which are easily customized to replicate a wide range of situations, are currently part of the curriculum in most medical schools. They are often customized to cover many aspects of a clinical encounter, and they offer medical students easy access to a range of medical situations. Human patient simulators allow students to engage in emotional and sensory learning. These interactive experiences foster critical thought and effective communication.

- Another way medical schools use new technology is with computer-aided instruction and "virtual" patients. Here, you'll apply newfound knowledge and skills via interactive web-based or software programs that simulate complex cases. Some advantages of computer-aided instruction are that it:

    o   Enables visualizing complex processes

    o   Allows independent exploration

    o   Offers easy access

    o   Costs relatively little

To learn more about the specific teaching methods of the medical schools you're interested in, please see the applicable school listing on the Medical School Admission Requirements™ website (*aamc.org/msar*).

Determining How You Want to Practice Medicine

Required courses. Clerkships. Electives. There's a lot occupying your time and energy as you advance through medical school. At the end of your third year and the beginning of your final year, you'll prepare to apply to residency programs. But before you can apply, you must make some serious decisions about how you want to practice medicine and identify the additional medical training that will prepare you for that work. All this career planning is commonly summarized as "choosing a specialty" and "applying for residency."

Choosing a Specialty

Choosing a medical specialty is one of the most significant decisions you'll make during medical school, and the process can be daunting. No one can prescribe which specialties are best for you. Making a good specialty decision requires you to be proactive. You'll likely begin the process of figuring out which specialties align with your interests, talents, and passions soon after you enter medical school.

The first step in choosing a specialty involves exploring what you want in your medical career. You can do this by:

- Observing and evaluating what you enjoy and what makes you happy across your experiences before and during medical school

- Objectively considering your career preferences using the Careers in Medicine® (CiM) self-assessments

- Engaging in specific activities that can help with the decision, such as shadowing physicians to learn about the work they do and find out whether you'll enjoy it

As a result of such efforts, you'll better understand your interests, values, skills, and other attributes, as well as your personal, educational, and career goals. This information will be most useful as you gain firsthand exposure to specialties during your clinical rotations, which occur in the third and final year of medical school. These rotations will be your most concentrated opportunity to "try on" different specialties. If by the start of your rotations you've already thoroughly considered who you are and what you want for your career, your rotations will provide much more insight for you.

Applying for Residency

Once you've chosen your specialty or specialties of interest, you must research and select residency programs in those specialties, then compete for a position in those programs. Much like the application process for medical school, you'll complete an application, craft a personal statement, and submit transcripts and letters of evaluation. An application service, such as the AAMC **Electronic Residency Application Service**® (ERAS®, *aamc.org/eras*), usually facilitates this process by electronically sending your application portfolio to your chosen residency programs. The application service(s) you use are determined by the specialty or specialties you're applying to (though ERAS is the application service that includes the most specialties and is used by the most applicants).

Once you've submitted your application portfolio to your chosen residency programs, these programs will review your materials and decide whether to invite you for an on-site interview. Once all interviews are complete, both residency applicants and individual programs rank their preferences and submit them to a matching service. The matching service runs an algorithm to compare the applicants' list of preferred programs with the programs' list of preferred applicants. After the algorithm runs, you'll learn if you've "matched" to a residency program.

The matching service that includes the most specialties and is used by the most applicants is the **National Resident Matching Program**® (NRMP®, *nrmp.org*), which runs its match the third week in March. That Friday—commonly known as Match Day—is met with great anticipation, as 17,000 medical school seniors learn where they'll spend the next several years of training. (These 17,000 students are the graduates of medical schools that grant the MD degree. In addition, 18,000 graduates of osteopathic schools [those granting the DO degree] and Canadian and international medical schools compete for residency program assignments through the NRMP. To learn more about ERAS and NRMP, go to *aamc.org/ eras* and *nrmp.org*. There is also a specific match solely for students at DO-granting schools through the AOA Intern/Resident Registration program. For more information, go to *natmatch.com/aoairp*.)

You can view live-streaming sessions of Match Day ceremonies at many medical schools. Look for links posted on Facebook (*facebook.com/aamcpremed*) and Twitter (*@AAMCPreMed*) for more details. Other match programs commonly used by students include (but aren't limited to) the San Francisco Residency and Fellowship Matching Services (*sfmatch.org*) and Military Graduate Medical Education (*militarygme.org*).

Getting Help

Determining which career path is right for you, as well as navigating the specialty choice and residency application and match process, is a lot for someone to manage alone—and you shouldn't. Many resources and people (including your student affairs office, mentors, and advisors) are available to help you make wise decisions about your future career.

One key resource is **Careers in Medicine** (CiM), a career planning program created by the AAMC and available to medical students and medical schools. Through its website (*aamc.org/cim*), CiM provides information, best practices, data, and tools to help you:

- Identify career goals

- Explore specialty and practice options

- Choose a specialty

- Select and apply to residency programs

- Learn to make good career decisions

Here are some examples of what the CiM website offers:

- Self-assessments that help you explore your interests, values, and skills so that you can identify specialties that might fit you well

- A database of clinical and research opportunities available to you during medical school

- Profiles of more than 120 specialties, including

    o   Descriptions of the work

    o   Salary and lifestyle information

    o   Workforce data

    o   Prerequisites and length of training for residency and fellowship programs

    o   Residency interview timing

    o   More than 1,000 links to additional specialty information

- Profiles of about 9,000 residency and fellowship programs and a tool to help you evaluate programs

- Information about various practice settings

- Lots of guidance and advice

For more information about how to access CiM, visit *aamc.org/cim*.

CiM works in conjunction with medical schools' career advising programs. Medical schools are required to provide advisors formally or informally to help students plan their academic and professional career. These services are often organized and delivered by the student affairs office or career center and can include workshops, specialty interest groups and panels, networking receptions, and other career-related resources and opportunities.

Sometime in your first year, your medical school will likely start talking to you about exploring your career options and planning your medical career as well as explaining the career-planning and career-advising services it offers. (If you'd like to start exploring your career sooner, contact your school's student affairs office.) Once your third year begins, your school will likely provide more intensive support by, for example, explaining the processes of and noting deadlines for choosing a specialty and applying for residency. This valuable information will come in various forms, including emails and in person from your student affairs office, your career services office, and your advisors.

Career planning will occur throughout your medical school experience, often within your curricular activities. As you complete your medical degree, faculty and advisors will be a source of trustworthy advice that will help guide you toward a satisfying career as a physician.

More Medical Training: Graduate Medical Education

Once you've graduated from medical school, you can claim the "doctor" title, but you can't yet practice medicine independently. You're required to progress from undergraduate medical education (that is, medical school) to graduate medical education (GME).

We won't go into detail about postgraduate work here, since you won't need the details until later. But, in a nutshell, the primary purpose of graduate medical education is to give medical school graduates the skills and knowledge they need to become competent, independent physicians in their desired specialty.

Table 3.2. U.S. Residents by Specialty, 2016–2017

Specialty	Number of U.S. Residents
Allergy and Immunology	279
Anesthesiology	5,591
Colon and Rectal Surgery	83
Dermatology	1,260
Emergency Medicine	5,916
Family Medicine	10,359
Hospice and Palliative Medicine	226
Internal Medicine	23,664
Medical Genetics	73
Neurological Surgery	1,337
Neurology	2,305
Nuclear Medicine	84
Obstetrics and Gynecology	5,061
Ophthalmology	1,349
Orthopedic Surgery	3,617
Otolaryngology	1,501
Pain Medicine	287
Pathology-Anatomic and Clinical	2,245
Pediatrics	8,661
Physical Medicine and Rehabilitation	1,268
Plastic Surgery	348
Plastic Surgery-Integrated*	672
Preventive Medicine	279
Psychiatry	5,153
Radiation Oncology	714
Radiology-Diagnostic	4,460
Sleep Medicine	132
Surgery-General	8,312
Thoracic Surgery	215
Thoracic Surgery-Integrated*	149
Urology	1,236

*The most popular subspecialties in 2016–2017 in internal medicine were cardiovascular disease (2,771), hematology and oncology (1,757), pulmonary disease and critical care medicine (1,677), gastroenterology (1,558), and nephrology (970).
**Integrated programs differ from subspecialty programs in that they include core surgical education.
Source: AAMC Data Book, 2017, for the 2016–2017 academic year, and the AAMC Careers in Medicine® program.

Residency and Fellowship Training

Residency training—the first level of GME—ranges in length from three to eight years (sometimes more) and is necessary for board certification (see Figure 3.2). Residency programs are conducted primarily in clinical settings (for example, in hospitals, outpatient clinics, community health centers, and physicians' offices) and require residents to participate fully in patient diagnoses and treatment. As a resident, you'll work under the supervision of physician faculty as you develop experience in your chosen specialty, become proficient with common and uncommon illnesses and conditions, attend conferences, teach less-experienced colleagues, and generally adjust to the demands of practicing medicine.

Just as medical schools vary, so do residency programs. Depending on the specialty you choose to pursue, you might complete a preliminary year of broad clinical training before focusing on your specialty. This practice is common in anesthesiology, dermatology, and radiology. In other fields, such as family medicine and pediatrics, you'll enter the specialty track directly. (Your medical school advisor and the Careers in Medicine program can provide more information as you approach this stage of your medical education.)

After residency training, you can continue your graduate medical education by completing fellowship training. This second level of GME usually prepares physicians to subspecialize, but some fellowships are for training in other areas, such as research or education administration.

Graduate medical education can be a challenging and rewarding stage of your career. Many physicians look back on their residency and fellowship years as a time when they gained invaluable lessons that they carry with them throughout their career.

Interprofessional Education

The delivery of medical care is increasingly a team-based, collaborative effort that includes doctors, nurses, pharmacists, physical therapists, and other health care providers. Caring for a patient effectively and efficiently depends on practitioners from all disciplines becoming familiar with one another's roles, perspectives, languages, and communication styles.

Because medical educators across the levels of medical education want to help you develop that knowledge and ability, your medical education is likely to involve some form of "interprofessional education." You'll learn to share resources, work as a unit, or participate in other activities that encourage interaction among various categories of health care providers. Through these exercises, you'll all become more adept and successful working as a team and, ultimately, be able to deliver higher-quality patient care.

Licensure and Certification: Ready to Practice Independently

All medical school graduates must demonstrate command of the same fundamental concepts before becoming licensed physicians. Physicians' mastery of these fundamentals is ensured through the standards of the **National Board of Medical Examiners** (NBME) and the **Federation of State Medical Boards** (FSMB). These two bodies jointly sponsor the **United States Medical Licensing Examination** (USMLE). This exam is the final assessment of your ability to assume independent responsibility for delivering medical care and is administered in three steps, each at a particular stage of medical education:

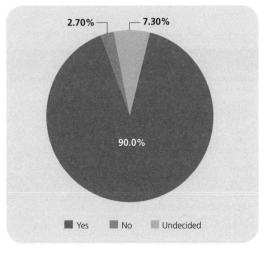

Figure 3.2. Medical school graduates' answers when asked whether they planned to become certified in a specific specialty.

2.70% 7.30%

90.0%

■ Yes   ■ No   ■ Undecided

Source: AAMC's 2017 Graduation Questionnaire (GQ).

- **Step 1:** Usually taken at the end of your second year of medical school, Step 1 tests whether you understand and can apply sciences basic to the practice of medicine. Its focus is on principles and systems of health, disease, and methods of therapy.

- **Step 2:** Many medical schools require you to take and pass Step 2 before you graduate. It's actually two tests in one—the first evaluates your clinical knowledge (CK) and the second your clinical skills (CS). Basically, Step 2 assesses your ability to provide patient care under supervision.

- **Step 3:** After you've completed your first year of residency training, you're eligible for Step 3— the concluding test that determines your readiness to apply your medical knowledge and clinical skills without supervision, with an emphasis on patient management in outpatient settings.

After you complete your educational and training programs and achieve passing scores on the USMLE, you can apply for licensure in any of the 50 states, 10 Canadian provinces, 3 U.S. territories, and the District of Columbia.

But … there is one additional step: certification. Although it's not required for medical practice, as licensure from a state or provincial medical board is, certification in a specialty is strongly encouraged (see Table 3.2). Physicians apply voluntarily for this additional credential, which is granted by the American Board of Medical Specialties (ABMS) and involves a comprehensive exam. (Those who have satisfied all ABMS requirements are certified and known as "diplomates" of the specialty board.) Most medical school graduates plan to become certified in a medical specialty (see Figure 3.2).

Continuing Medical Education: Lifelong Learning

Finally, as you likely have realized, your medical education will be a lifelong process. As medicine continues to advance and change, you'll be given the opportunity to learn new skills to stay current with exciting and innovative developments.

The fast pace of change in medicine makes continuing education essential, so most states require participation in accredited continuing medical education (CME) activities. Physicians participate in CME programs throughout their careers, ensuring that they stay up-to-date with the rapid advancements in their specialties and they maintain their clinical competence. Offered by medical schools, teaching hospitals, and professional organizations, these CME programs are reviewed by the **Accreditation Council for Continuing Medical Education** (ACCME) to ensure that high standards are achieved and upheld.

CME reflects a commitment to lifelong learning that's a hallmark of the medical profession. If you're interested in what your CME efforts will entail, go to *accme.org*.

 Worksheets at the end of chapters in this guide are available in fillable PDF format at *aamc.org/msar-resources*.

First things first: You do not need to know your medical specialty now—or even need to be thinking about it. However, many applicants envision themselves in a particular specialty before day one of medical school. These visions can often be tied to the shadowing or medically related volunteer experiences that many applicants participate in to help prepare for medical school. If you're one of these applicants, it likely means you're already familiar with one or more medical specialties.

Now, the second thing to keep in mind: Changing your mind about what type of physician you want to be is not a sign that you're less committed to the profession. We know from responses to the AAMC Matriculating Student Questionnaire and Graduation Questionnaire that most medical students are either undecided about their specialty preference or change their minds about their specialty preference over the course of medical school. It's natural and expected that your choices will evolve as you progress through medical school and gain new educational and clinical experiences. So, keep your options open to allow for something amazing you have yet to encounter to inspire you and change your life. And enjoy the reprieve of waiting a little while to finalize your specialty choice.

That being said, if you're an applicant with some exposure to specialties before medical school, you may find it helpful to keep a journal or notes about your experiences while they're fresh in your mind, which you can use once you enter medical school and begin the Careers in Medicine program (*aamc.org/cim*). You'll likely find it helpful to refer back to these notes once you've matriculated and as you progress through medical school.

Here are some prompts to help you consider your specialty experiences:

- Do you have a specialty or specialties in mind? _____

    _____

- What is your experience with that specialty? _____

    _____

- Have you shadowed in that specialty with different physicians or in different settings?_____

    _____

- Have you shadowed in more than one specialty? If so, list here: _____

    _____

- Take a moment to compare your experiences. Write down how they were similar and different and how you felt about each. _____

    _____

You can also visit your school's career center for more guidance about exploring medical careers. A career center may be able to help you find shadowing and other opportunities that can expose you to career options. You could also speak with people who have already completed any experiences you're considering.

A note about shadowing: In recent years, due to the Health Insurance Portability and Accountability Act, or HIPAA, it may be more difficult to obtain permission to shadow a physician. There are programs that facilitate paid experiences domestically and abroad. They can be quite expensive. Be certain to check with your prehealth advising office to see if they have experience with a particular program to make sure it's legitimate and safe.

For more information about shadowing, lab, and volunteer experiences, see:

- **Shadowing a Doctor**—*students-residents.aamc.org/applying-medical-school/article/howgetlabexperience*

- **Getting Lab Experience**—*aamc.org/students/aspiring/experience/280610/labexperience.html*

- **Finding Health Care–Related Volunteer Opportunities**—*students-residents.aamc.org/applying-medical-school/article/finding-health-care-related-volunteer-opportunities*

CHAPTER 4

Building Toward Greater Diversity

> *As a student who completed the AAMC Summer Medical and Dental Education Program, I was exposed to the need for diversity in the physician workforce early on in my undergraduate years. It was important for me to choose a medical school that understood that the concept of diversity in medicine was an expansive one. Diversity does not just mean ethnic or racial variation; it also means diversity of thought, language, education, gender, and socioeconomic status.*
>
> *Through my work with immigrants who are underserved and speak English as a second language, I learned about the need for physicians to have experience with diverse populations. Many of my Bangladeshi-American family members feel that physicians don't understand their culture, language, and customs. Non–English speaking populations often feel that their voices are not heard and that the actual story behind their illness gets miscommunicated by the translator.*
>
> *It is imperative that American medical schools produce culturally competent physicians who understand diversity in medicine. Otherwise, patients may feel that physicians were quick to make judgments and feel unsatisfied with the level of care. Physicians who understand the patient's language, culture, religion, gender identity, and sexual orientation create meaningful relationships with the patients and make them feel comfortable. Physicians who are well equipped to handle the diverse country we live in will be able to change the medical care of the future by delivering high-quality, personalized medical care.*

Subha Hanif
MD Candidate
Michigan State University College
of Human Medicine
Class of 2019

Defining Diversity

When people hear the word *diversity*, many probably think in terms of race and ethnicity. And while it is certainly important to have more racial and ethnic minority populations represented in medicine, the concept of diversity is much more expansive.

Diversity refers to the richness of human differences—socioeconomic status, race, ethnicity, language, nationality, sex, gender identity, sexual orientation, religion, geography, disability, age, and individual aspects such as personality, learning styles, and life experiences. Let's look at diversity through the lens of available AAMC data.

- **First, consider race and ethnicity.** While diversity extends beyond this particular characteristic, it remains a critical component. The data show, for example, that only 8.2% of applicants are black or African-American, 6.2% are Hispanic or Latino, and 0.2% are American Indian or Alaska Native. (See Figure 4.1.)

- **What about family income?**
  This is an area of great imbalance. Parental income of students entering medical school skews heavily to the upper range, with a median income of $125,000. (That's almost double the estimated U.S. median family income of $56,516 reported by the U.S. Census Bureau.) Looking at it from another angle, more than one in five students comes from a home in which their parents earn $250,000 or more a year. (See Figure 4.2.)

- **Another perspective—gender.**
  On the surface, it appears that male and female applicants are fairly equal in number, but there are instances where that's not the case. You'll see, for example, in Figure 4.1, that there are significantly fewer black or African-American male applicants. The AAMC recently published *Altering the Course: Black Males in Medicine* to better understand this trend and explore solutions (*aamc.org/blackmalesinmed*).

- **Benefits of diversity extend beyond education.** Increased diversity brings with it benefits that extend beyond the classroom. Research has shown that diversity in the physician workforce contributes to increased access to health care. Diversity among clinician scientists has been linked to an increase in research dedicated to diseases that disproportionately affect racial and ethnic minorities.

Figure 4.1. Applicants to U.S. medical schools, by race, ethnicity, and sex, 2017–2018.

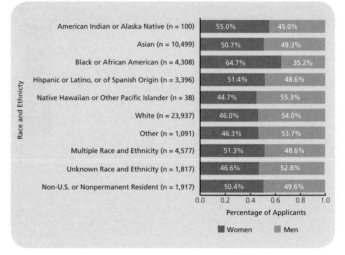

Note: *Applicants who did not report sex were excluded. The Multiple Race and Ethnicity category includes those who selected more than one race and/or ethnicity response.*
Source: *AAMC Data Warehouse, Applicant Matriculant File, as of May 2018.*

Figure 4.2. Parental income of entering medical students, 2017.

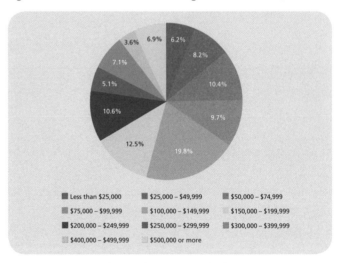

Source: *AAMC's 2017 Matriculating Student Questionnaire (MSQ).*

AAMC Programs and Resources

The AAMC is committed to improving health for all. Considering the benefits that diversity offers, the AAMC is engaged in a number of programs and initiatives designed to help increase diversity to include students from a broad range of backgrounds. While these programs are open to all students, they are sensitive to the challenges and needs of individuals from groups underrepresented in medicine. Here are some of these initiatives.

Career Fairs and Enrichment Programs

Medical schools throughout the country provide various programs and resources designed to recruit students and prepare them for medical education. Some of these programs are held during the school year, others in the summer. They are designed for high school students, college students, and those who already have completed undergraduate study. It's a good idea to explore the local medical school's website to see what opportunities may be available.

The AAMC sponsors several programs:

- **Minority Student Medical Career Fair.** This event is typically held each fall in conjunction with Learn Serve Lead: The AAMC Annual Meeting. Students are encouraged to come and explore the possibilities in medicine and science. College and high school students, parents, prehealth advisors, school administrators, and any others interested in pursuing a career in medicine and science can meet diversity affairs and admissions officers from U.S. medical schools and other health professions schools to discuss medical school preparation, enrichment programs, admissions policies and procedures, financial aid, and more. Attendees can also participate in interactive medical and health activities and workshops. The AAMC also hosts other career fairs in conjunction with meetings for student affairs and graduate education. Information about these events is available at *aamc.org/medicalcareerfair*.

- **Summer Health Professions Education Program (SHPEP).** The Robert Wood Johnson Foundation's Summer Health Professions Education Program is a free, six-week academic enrichment program for college freshmen and sophomores interested in careers in medicine, dentistry, pharmacy, nursing, public health, physician assistant, optometry, and physical therapy. Components of the program include science- and quantitative-based courses, learning and study skills seminars, career development activities, clinical experiences, and a financial planning workshop. Funded by the Robert Wood Johnson Foundation and offered at 13 U.S. institutions across the nation, the program includes a stipend, housing, and meals. For additional information, visit *shpep.org*.

- **Medical School Virtual Fair.** The AAMC also hosts a virtual medical school fair in February. This free event gives attendees a chance to speak with medical school admissions officers and AAMC content experts about admission- and medical-school-related topics, including admissions policies, financial aid, the MCAT exam, and American Medical College Application Service® (AMCAS®) applications.

Aspiring Docs®—An AAMC Resource to Increase Diversity in Medicine

Having a diverse workforce of physicians and scientists is essential to providing the best care and improving the health of all.

The AAMC's Aspiring Docs® website provides resources and inspiration to help you get started on your path to medicine. The website includes inspiring stories from medical students and doctors about how they overcame challenges, videos of medical students answering questions from applicants, and one-page fact sheets to help you get started as you prepare to apply. To see what other applicants are saying about being a premed, and to read what medical students and residents are doing every day, follow the Aspiring Docs Diaries blog (*aspiringdocsdiaries.org*). You can even email *aspiringdocs@aamc.org* if you'd like to submit a blog post!

Aspiring Docs offers the most reliable tools and information to anyone considering a career in medicine. To access the growing library of information and resources, visit *aamc.org/aspiringdocs.*

Additional AAMC Resources

The AAMC also offers a wide variety of publications, online tools, and other information at the Minorities in Medicine website at *aamc.org/students/minorities* and the Diversity and Inclusion website at *aamc.org/diversity.* Among the resources you will find are:

Medical Students with Disabilities: Resources to Enhance Accessibility. This guide informs users about current resources available to medical schools as they accept and matriculate a growing number of medical students with a wide range of disabilities. Specifically, there is an emphasis in this publication on the assistive technologies available for medical students. You can order a copy of this guide at *members.aamc.org/eweb/DynamicPage.aspx?webcode=PubHome.*

Enrichment Programs Online. This site includes a free database to help students locate summer enrichment programs on medical school campuses. You can search by school, state, region, area of focus, and length of program. Go to *services.aamc.org/summerprograms* to explore programs of interest.

Medical Minority Applicant Registry (Med-MAR). During the MCAT registration, students who are either economically disadvantaged or from racial and ethnic groups that are historically underrepresented in medicine can select the Medical Minority Applicant Registry (Med-MAR) option to be included in the registry. This web-based program provides medical schools with basic biographical information and MCAT scores of registered examinees, thereby giving institutions opportunities to enhance their diversity efforts. Go to *aamc.org/medmar* for more information.

For information about the definition of "underrepresented" in medicine, visit *aamc.org/urm.*

Fee Assistance Program. The AAMC believes that the cost of applying to medical school should not be an insurmountable barrier. Its Fee Assistance Program is available to students whose financial limitations would otherwise prevent them from taking the MCAT exam or applying to medical school.

Details about the Fee Assistance Program can be found at *aamc.org/students/applying/fap* and in Chapter 7 of this guide.

Data About Applicants, Matriculants, and Graduates. The AAMC also collects and presents detailed data about medical students from different racial and ethnic groups, most of which are available online free of charge on the AAMC website (and a good deal of which are included in this guide). (See also Table 4.1 at the end of this chapter.) Several resources are likely to be of interest:

- A large collection of data about medical school applicants, matriculants, and graduates is available on the AAMC website at *aamc.org/facts.*

- The AAMC publication *Diversity in Medical Education, Facts & Figures 2016* provides race and ethnicity data on medical school applicants, accepted applicants, matriculants, enrollment, graduates, and faculty. You can access the full text without charge at *aamcdiversityfactsandfigures2016.org.*

- Data on medical school faculty, including information by self-identification, can be found at *aamc.org/data/facultyroster/reports.*

School Programs and Resources

Just as the AAMC is committed to diversity and inclusion, colleges and medical schools are also invested in making medical education accessible to all. Explore these other resources as well.

Premedical School Programs at Undergraduate Colleges. Prehealth advisors have an abundance of information and data at their fingertips. Not only can they help you with the application process and refer you to appropriate contacts, they also know about programs that students from underrepresented groups and disadvantaged backgrounds have found useful. If your college has a prehealth advisor (and the majority of them do), make sure you take advantage of this valuable resource.

Medical School Websites. In addition to the individual profiles in the Medical School Admission Requirements™ website, you'll want to explore the medical school websites for information on their diversity programs and resources. Go to *aamc.org/medicalschools* for a listing of all U.S. and Canadian MD-granting medical schools and links to their websites.

Medical School Diversity Affairs Representatives. Other invaluable resources are medical school diversity affairs representatives. These individuals are dedicated to increasing diversity among medical schools at their institutions and are an excellent source of information for applicants (or potential applicants). You can get the name of the diversity affairs contacts at any U.S. medical school through the Directory of Diversity Affairs Representatives database. It's searchable by name, location, and institution, and it's available at *members. aamc.org/eweb/DynamicPage.aspx?site=AAMC&webcod e=AAMCOrgSearchResult&orgtype=Medical%20School*

Contact information is also available within each medical school profile on the Medical School Admission Requirements website at *aamc.org/msar*.

Financial Assistance for Medical School. Don't let the cost of medical school deter you from your dreams. As you'll learn in Chapter 10, more than four-fifths of medical students across the country receive some form of financial assistance. Medical schools—both public and private—work hard to offer a variety of financial aid plans to ensure that capable students are not denied access to their institutions because of financial limitations. In addition to discussing possibilities for assistance with the financial aid officer at the medical schools that interest you, you should familiarize yourself with general information about financing a medical education by reading the relevant material in this book and reviewing the wealth of information about loans (and other programs) at *aamc.org/first*.

Programs at Medical Schools. Once you've enrolled in medical school, you'll find that a variety of academic and personal support programs is available to you. These programs help students from various backgrounds to successfully complete their medical studies, with the ultimate goal of increasing diversity among physicians entering careers in patient care, teaching, and research and eliminating racial and ethnic disparities in health care.

For those who wish to explore the benefits of diversity, we suggest the following essential readings:

Antonio AL, Chang MJ, Hakuta K, Kenny DA, Levin S, Milem JF. Effects of racial diversity on complex thinking in college students. *Psychological Science*. 2004;15:507–510.

Denson N, Chang M. Racial diversity matters: The impact of diversity-related student engagement and institutional context. *American Educational Research Journal*. 2009;46(2):322–353.

Gurin P. The compelling need for diversity in higher education: Expert testimony in Gratz, et al. v. Bollinger, et al. *Michigan Journal of Race and Law*. 1999;5:363–425.

Saha S, Guiton G, Wimmers PF, Wilkerson L. Student body racial and ethnic composition and diversity-related outcomes in US medical schools. *JAMA*. 2008;300:1135–1145.

Smith DG. *Diversity's Promise for Higher Education: Making It Work*. Baltimore, MD: The Johns Hopkins University Press; 2009.

Smith DG and Associates. *Diversity Works: The Emerging Picture of How Students Benefit*. Washington, DC: Association of American Colleges and Universities; 1997.

Whitla DK, Orfield G, Silen W, Teperow C, Howard C, Reede J. Educational benefit of diversity in medical school: A survey of students. *Academic Medicine*. 2003;78:460–466.

No Advisor? Contact the NAAHP for Help

If your institution does not have a prehealth advisor, you can contact the **National Association of Advisors for the Health Professions** (NAAHP). There, you'll find a list of NAAHP members who have volunteered to help students without access to a prehealth advisor from a distance. Learn more about what prehealth advisors do and how to locate one at *naahp.org/StudentResources/FindanAdvisor.aspx*.

Table 4.1. Matriculants, by Medical School, Race, and Ethnicity, 2017*

State	School	Hispanic or Latino	Asian	American Indian or Alaska Native	Black	Native Hawaiian/OPI	White	Other	Unduplicated Total
AL	Alabama	4	24	6	7	0	150	3	186
AL	South Alabama	1	8	1	9	0	57	0	74
AR	Arkansas	12	14	2	6	0	145	3	173
AZ	Arizona	29	28	5	7	0	71	5	132
AZ	Arizona Phoenix	11	17	0	6	0	51	4	83
CA	California Northstate	7	44	0	1	1	37	8	90
CA	Loma Linda	16	61	0	12	1	77	2	168
CA	Southern Cal-Keck	28	71	0	17	2	63	10	184
CA	Stanford	12	40	0	9	2	31	0	93
CA	UC Berkeley/SF Joint Prog	3	9	1	1	0	7	0	16
CA	UC Davis	32	36	2	10	0	38	10	110
CA	UC Irvine	18	41	0	4	0	43	8	104
CA	UC Riverside	11	22	0	6	0	21	9	60
CA	UC San Diego	18	49	1	6	0	77	2	134
CA	UC San Francisco	29	52	0	18	1	60	13	149
CA	UCLA Drew	12	0	1	13	0	0	1	24
CA	UCLA-Geffen	29	55	3	19	1	55	8	151
CO	Colorado	24	34	10	9	2	130	7	182
CT	Connecticut	9	21	1	13	0	61	1	100
CT	Quinnipiac-Netter	4	28	1	9	2	45	9	90
CT	Yale	7	40	3	14	0	35	4	104
DC	George Washington	18	51	1	16	1	104	7	177
DC	Georgetown	10	38	1	13	0	133	5	196
DC	Howard	7	15	1	77	0	11	1	112
FL	FIU-Wertheim	44	34	2	13	1	46	5	126
FL	Florida	22	23	1	14	0	90	7	135
FL	Florida Atlantic-Schmidt	8	4	1	8	0	43	3	63
FL	Florida State	15	20	0	19	0	74	4	120
FL	Miami-Miller	35	56	1	20	1	94	5	196
FL	UCF	10	33	1	7	0	71	7	120
FL	USF-Morsani	20	57	1	12	0	107	5	183
GA	Emory	7	30	0	12	0	90	3	136
GA	MC Georgia Augusta	18	63	0	35	0	126	10	230
GA	Mercer	5	20	0	4	0	94	3	122
GA	Morehouse	5	15	1	65	0	11	2	92
HI	Hawaii-Burns	4	57	1	0	8	12	1	70
IA	Iowa-Carver	13	22	2	8	1	117	3	152
IL	Chicago Med Franklin	8	76	0	7	1	97	6	191
IL	Chicago-Pritzker	7	24	1	16	0	54	1	91
IL	Illinois	60	95	2	27	0	146	15	317
IL	Loyola-Stritch	19	37	3	26	1	77	10	159
IL	Northwestern-Feinberg	16	58	0	11	1	78	3	163
IL	Rush	5	37	0	10	0	86	2	136
IL	Southern Illinois	0	7	0	7	0	57	1	71
IN	Indiana	50	57	1	32	0	227	7	352
KS	Kansas	12	23	2	7	0	171	7	211
KY	Kentucky	2	13	0	5	0	109	1	136
KY	Louisville	4	20	0	15	0	113	4	156
LA	LSU New Orleans	9	25	0	8	0	159	2	197
LA	LSU Shreveport	5	12	1	5	1	100	4	124
LA	Tulane	5	47	3	11	2	130	6	191
MA	Boston	34	54	1	3	0	96	8	190
MA	Harvard	15	51	1	10	1	72	10	165
MA	Massachusetts	3	40	1	11	0	91	7	150
MA	Tufts	16	51	4	13	3	133	9	211
MD	Johns Hopkins	8	50	0	6	1	52	2	118
MD	Maryland	8	53	0	12	0	87	6	161
MD	Uniformed Services-Hébert	14	30	2	10	2	125	4	171
MI	Central Michigan	9	11	0	5	0	72	7	101
MI	Michigan	14	38	0	14	0	113	5	172

(continued)

State	School	Hispanic or Latino	Asian	American Indian or Alaska Native	Black	Native Hawaiian/OPI	White	Other	Unduplicated Total
MI	Michigan State	10	29	0	19	0	113	15	177
MI	Oakland Beaumont	2	40	2	7	0	66	11	125
MI	Wayne State	24	57	4	33	0	163	38	286
MI	Western Michigan-Stryker	4	22	1	1	0	46	4	72
MN	Mayo	4	11	2	2	2	33	3	51
MN	Minnesota	9	22	10	24	0	172	3	229
MO	Missouri Columbia	4	19	1	5	0	79	1	104
MO	Missouri Kansas City	6	43	3	7	0	53	2	120
MO	Saint Louis	6	59	1	21	1	89	4	180
MO	Washington U St Louis	8	40	3	8	0	66	0	123
MS	Mississippi	5	16	0	10	0	115	4	145
NC	Duke	7	30	3	19	1	64	2	119
NC	East Carolina-Brody	3	11	2	9	0	52	3	80
NC	North Carolina	9	27	3	27	0	119	6	180
NC	Wake Forest	8	23	0	17	0	82	6	129
ND	North Dakota	2	6	8	1	0	64	5	78
NE	Creighton	7	33	0	1	2	118	7	154
NE	Nebraska	6	11	0	6	0	106	2	126
NH	Dartmouth-Geisel	10	21	3	6	1	53	3	92
NJ	Cooper Rowan	5	20	0	17	0	44	6	88
NJ	Rutgers New Jersey	16	76	0	23	0	65	11	178
NJ	Rutgers-RW Johnson	11	51	0	14	0	81	5	160
NM	New Mexico	38	14	4	2	0	52	6	103
NV	Nevada Reno	9	16	0	3	0	42	4	68
NY	Albany	12	51	1	9	0	66	5	134
NY	Buffalo-Jacobs	16	40	1	7	0	89	4	149
NY	CUNY	10	23	1	25	0	22	0	69
NY	Columbia	19	35	0	13	1	83	3	151
NY	Cornell-Weill	9	35	1	5	2	51	4	106
NY	Einstein	14	58	1	7	0	101	8	183
NY	Hofstra Northwell	9	32	0	10	0	52	3	99
NY	Mount Sinai-Icahn	14	40	0	16	0	81	3	140
NY	New York Medical	16	64	2	14	0	120	9	213
NY	New York University	15	40	0	11	0	69	1	129
NY	Rochester	10	29	1	13	0	54	3	104
NY	SUNY Downstate	10	75	0	16	0	86	9	190
NY	SUNY Upstate	11	31	1	19	1	90	8	160
NY	Stony Brook	15	46	0	6	1	66	3	132
OH	Case Western Reserve	11	80	0	13	0	110	7	216
OH	Cincinnati	13	27	1	12	0	127	4	170
OH	Northeast Ohio	1	51	2	8	2	81	8	148
OH	Ohio State	20	46	2	29	1	114	10	199
OH	Toledo	3	40	0	3	0	122	6	174
OH	Wright State-Boonshoft	7	11	0	19	0	72	0	108
OK	Oklahoma	11	32	13	4	0	123	2	165
OR	Oregon	10	28	2	6	2	111	6	153
PA	Commonwealth	9	17	1	2	1	82	2	108
PA	Drexel	15	73	0	17	0	152	18	260
PA	Jefferson-Kimmel	9	68	0	9	0	183	5	266
PA	Penn State	9	33	1	15	1	90	3	144
PA	Pennsylvania-Perelman	19	35	0	18	1	76	4	146
PA	Pittsburgh	7	27	0	15	0	102	1	148
PA	Temple-Katz	25	60	0	16	0	122	5	206
PR	Caribe	69	1	0	0	0	4	0	70
PR	Ponce	78	1	1	2	0	11	1	83
PR	Puerto Rico	112	0	0	1	0	4	0	112
PR	San Juan Bautista	56	3	0	0	0	10	1	63
RI	Brown-Alpert	18	39	0	15	0	83	1	144
SC	MU South Carolina	11	16	3	19	0	134	5	176
SC	South Carolina	0	11	0	8	0	77	2	97
SC	South Carolina Greenville	7	7	1	5	0	84	3	103

(continued)

Table 4.1. Matriculants, by Medical School, Race, and Ethnicity, 2017* *(continued)*

State	School	Hispanic or Latino	Asian	American Indian or Alaska Native	Black	Native Hawaiian/OPI	White	Other	Unduplicated Total
SD	South Dakota-Sanford	2	2	1	0	0	63	1	66
TN	East Tennessee-Quillen	0	6	0	1	0	62	2	68
TN	Meharry	8	5	5	92	0	7	2	108
TN	Tennessee	4	30	0	5	0	134	4	170
TN	Vanderbilt	6	17	1	12	0	57	3	89
TX	Baylor	25	67	0	9	1	98	1	186
TX	Texas A & M	17	72	1	5	0	99	3	183
TX	Texas Tech	26	46	1	10	0	101	1	180
TX	Texas Tech-Foster	35	24	0	3	0	57	0	103
TX	UT Austin-Dell	7	9	1	3	0	37	0	50
TX	UT HSC San Antonio	39	70	1	14	1	121	5	215
TX	UT Houston-McGovern	42	65	3	20	0	134	5	240
TX	UT Medical Branch	39	77	0	16	1	121	4	230
TX	UT Rio Grande Valley	23	9	1	6	0	28	3	55
TX	UT Southwestern	33	99	2	22	0	94	8	230
UT	Utah	3	16	0	1	1	105	2	125
VA	Eastern Virginia	5	44	4	6	0	101	2	151
VA	Virginia	18	28	3	21	0	97	6	156
VA	Virginia Commonwealth	11	93	0	4	0	104	9	216
VA	Virginia Tech Carilion	3	14	1	2	0	24	2	42
VT	Vermont	14	22	0	4	1	81	6	117
WA	U Washington	14	45	4	10	1	212	9	270
WI	MC Wisconsin	19	53	0	11	1	187	8	261
WI	Wisconsin	9	42	5	9	1	117	4	170
WV	Marshall-Edwards	1	10	1	4	0	67	4	83
WV	West Virginia	7	13	0	2	0	92	3	110

*Data are not reflective of the number of individuals in each demographic category, but rather the number of times a particular race or ethnic category was selected. One individual can self-identify with multiple groups.
Source: AAMC Data Warehouse: Applicant and Matriculant File as of November 22, 2017.

Worksheets at the end of chapters in this guide are available in fillable PDF format at *aamc.org/msar-resources*.

Use this worksheet to identify programs you may be eligible for. Many programs primarily sponsored by medical schools are available to students across the United States. You can start searching at *services.aamc.org/summerprograms* and *ExploreHealthCareers.org*, and then use this worksheet to figure out your options.

Before the Application Process

For example: Summer Health Professions Education Program (SHPEP)

- Description: Six-week academic enrichment program that offers students both academic and career experiences that will support their dental or medical school career preparation. For more Information, go to *shpep.org*.

- Eligibility: _____

- Which academic year(s) would I be eligible to participate?: _____

- When am I eligible to apply?: _____   • Application deadline: _____

- Accepts out-of-state?: ❏ Yes   ❏ No   ❏ Other: _____

- Application requirements: _____

_____

During the Application Process

For example: Medical Minority Applicant Registry (Med-MAR)

- Description: During the MCAT registration, students who are either economically disadvantaged or from racial and ethnic groups that are historically underrepresented in medicine can select the Medical Minority Applicant Registry (Med-MAR). This web-based program provides medical schools with basic biographical information and MCAT scores of registered examinees, thereby giving them opportunities to enhance their diversity efforts. For more information, go to *aamc.org/medmar*.

- Eligibility: _____

- Which academic year(s) would I be eligible to participate?: _____

- When am I eligible to apply?: _____   • Application deadline: _____

- Accepts out-of-state? ❏ Yes   ❏ No   ❏ Other: _____

- Application requirements: _____

_____

During the Application Process

Program: _____

- Description: _____

_____

- Eligibility: _____

- Which academic year(s) would I be eligible to participate?: _____

- When am I eligible to apply?: _____   • Application deadline: _____

- Accepts out-of-state? ❏ Yes   ❏ No   ❏ Other: _____

- Application requirements: _____

_____

CHAPTER 5

All About the MCAT® Exam

Preparing for the MCAT exam was a challenging yet fulfilling experience. Coming from a disadvantaged background and having no experience with standardized testing, the odds of succeeding were against me. I took the test more than once, learning from my mistakes and improving every time. In the end, my perseverance allowed me to do well on the exam and get into medical school.

I developed many skills while preparing for the MCAT exam, from time management skills to study habits and work-life-balance skills. One of the most important things I learned is that different study methods work for different people. It took time and troubleshooting to optimize my study strategy. One of the hardest things was being consistent and disciplined with my study schedule. I learned how to efficiently manage my time. With those new skills, I developed a plan that allowed me to do well.

I would recommend that you start studying well in advance for the MCAT exam and approaching the test with the goal of taking it only once. Don't set yourself up for failure by anticipating not doing well; instead, prepare yourself as much as possible to accomplish your goal. I was working a full-time job and studying 20 hours a week, but I also scheduled time to relax, exercise, and be with family. Looking back at my experience, I can say that it was all worth it.

Munir H. Buhaya
MD Candidate
University of Texas McGovern
Medical School at Houston
Class of 2021

The Role of the MCAT® Exam

Simply put, the MCAT exam helps admissions officers identify which students are likely to succeed in medical school. That's done by identifying those students who not only have a basic knowledge of the natural, behavioral, and social sciences—which provides the foundation necessary in the early years of medical school—but also those with strong critical analysis and reasoning skills.

It can be argued that college grades essentially do the same thing. But because an "A" at one school is not necessarily equivalent to an "A" at another, admissions officers don't have a "standard measure" against which to evaluate students. The MCAT exam fills that void. As a result, virtually every medical school in the United States, and many in Canada, requires applicants to submit recent MCAT scores.

Admissions officers look at MCAT scores in conjunction with your grades and with many other selection factors, including those related to your experiences and personal attributes, when making their decisions.

Using all these components, medical school admissions committees are able to substantially increase their success in predicting who will be successful in medical school.

Application programs and institutions that use MCAT scores include:

- American Medical College Application Service® (AMCAS®)
- American Association of Colleges of Osteopathic Medicine Application Service (AACOMAS)
- Texas Medical and Dental Schools Application Service (TMDSAS)
- Ontario Medical School Application Service (OMSAS)
- Other Canadian medical schools requiring MCAT scores
- American Association of Colleges of Podiatric Medicine Application Service (AACPM)
- Veterinary Medical College Application Service (VMCAS)
- Schools of Public Health Application Service (SOPHAS)

Eligibility

You're eligible to take the MCAT exam if you plan to apply to a health professions program, including:

- MD-granting
- DO-granting
- Podiatric (DPM)
- Veterinary medicine (DVM)
- Any other health-related program that will accept MCAT exam results to satisfy a test score admissions requirement

When you register, you'll be required to sign a statement verifying your intention to apply to a health professions school.

International Students

If you're an international student, you're welcome to take the MCAT exam, provided that you meet the eligibility requirements. If you're in an MBBS (bachelor of medicine/bachelor of surgery) degree program or hold the MBBS degree, you may register for the MCAT exam without seeking special permission.

How the Exam Is Structured

There are four multiple-choice test sections:

- Biological and Biochemical Foundations of Living Systems
- Chemical and Physical Foundations of Biological Systems
- Psychological, Social, and Biological Foundations of Behavior
- Critical Analysis and Reasoning Skills

The first three sections listed are organized around foundational concepts in the natural, behavioral, and social sciences. They reflect current research about the most effective ways for students to learn and use science, emphasizing deep knowledge of the most important scientific concepts.

Science education leaders say that some of the most important foundational concepts in the sciences ask students to integrate and analyze information from different disciplines. In that vein, questions in these sections will ask you to combine your scientific knowledge from multiple disciplines with your scientific inquiry and reasoning skills. On these three sections of the exam, you'll be asked to demonstrate four different scientific inquiry and reasoning skills:

- Knowledge of scientific concepts and principles

- Scientific reasoning and problem solving

- Reasoning about the design and execution of research

- Data-based and statistical reasoning

The fourth section, Critical Analysis and Reasoning Skills, will be similar to many of the verbal reasoning tests you've taken in your academic career. It includes passages and questions that test your ability to comprehend and analyze what you read. This section asks you to read and think about passages from a wide range of disciplines in the humanities and social sciences, including population health, ethics and philosophy, and studies of diverse cultures. Passages are followed by a series of questions that lead you through the process of comprehending, analyzing, and reasoning about the material you've read. This section was developed specifically to measure the analytical and reasoning skills you'll need to be successful in medical school.

What the Exam Measures

The different sections of the MCAT exam are carefully designed to test the concepts and skills most needed by entering medical students.

The Biological and Biochemical Foundations of Living Systems and the Chemical and Physical Foundations of Biological Systems sections are designed to:

- Test introductory-level biology, organic and inorganic chemistry, and physics concepts taught in yearlong courses

- Test biochemistry concepts at the level taught in many colleges and universities in first-semester biochemistry courses

- Test cellular and molecular biology topics at the level taught in many colleges and universities in introductory biology sequences and first-semester biochemistry courses

- Target basic research methods and statistics concepts described by many baccalaureate faculty as important to success in introductory science courses

- Have you demonstrate your scientific inquiry and reasoning, research methods, and statistics skills, as applied to the natural sciences

The Psychological, Social, and Biological Foundations of Behavior section is designed to:

- Test your knowledge and use of the concepts in psychology, sociology, and biology that provide a solid foundation for learning about the behavioral and sociocultural determinants of health in medical school

- Target concepts taught at many colleges and universities in first-semester psychology and sociology courses

- Target biology concepts that relate to mental processes and behavior that are taught at many colleges and universities in introductory biology

- Target basic research methods and statistics concepts described by many baccalaureate faculty as important to success in introductory science courses and described in many introductory psychology and sociology courses

- Have you demonstrate your scientific inquiry and reasoning, research methods, and statistics skills, as applied to the social and behavioral sciences

The Critical Analysis and Reasoning Skills section is designed to:

- Test your comprehension, analysis, and reasoning skills by asking you to critically analyze information provided in reading passages

- Include content from ethics, philosophy, studies of diverse cultures, population health, and a wide range of social sciences and humanities disciplines

- Provide you with all the information you need to answer questions in the passages

MCAT Scores

You'll receive five scores from your MCAT exam: one for each of the four sections and one combined, total score. The MCAT exam is not graded on a curve; it's equated. The equating process compensates for small differences in difficulty between test forms and ensures that scores have the same meaning no matter when you take the exam or what test form you get. Below is the information you'll receive in your score report.

Section Scores

Each of the four sections—Biological and Biochemical Foundations of Living Systems; Chemical and Physical Foundations of Biological Systems; Psychological, Social, and Biological Foundations of Behavior; and Critical Analysis and Reasoning Skills—is scored from a low of 118 to a high of 132, with a midpoint of 125. You'll receive a score for each of the four sections. (Figure 5.1 shows a sample score report.)

Total Score

Your scores for the four sections are combined to create your total score. The total score ranges from 472 to 528. The midpoint is 500.

For example, if you scored 127 on the Biological and Biochemical Foundations of Living Systems section; 124 on the Chemical and Physical Foundations of Biological Systems section; 127 on the Psychological, Social, and Biological Foundations of Behavior section; and 123 on the Critical Analysis and Reasoning Skills section, your total score would be 501.

Confidence Bands

Like other standardized tests, the MCAT exam is an imperfect measure of what test takers know and can do. Examinees' scores can be affected by factors like fatigue, test anxiety, and distractions during the test. But then again, an examinee's score might be boosted if they were recently exposed to some of the topics included on the exam. The inclusion of the confidence bands is meant to remind admissions officers not to overemphasize small differences in test scores.

Percentile Ranks

The percentile ranks show how you scored relative to other MCAT examinees. You'll receive a percentile rank for each individual section score and for your overall total score. Each percentile rank represents

Figure 5.1. Sample MCAT score report.

Most Recent Exam

Section	Score	Confidence Band [1]	Percentile Rank of Score [2]	Score Profile [3]
Chemical and Physical Foundations of Biological Systems	124	123◇125	45%	
Critical Analysis and Reasoning Skills	123	122◇124	33%	
Biological and Biochemical Foundations of Living Systems	127	126◇128	77%	
Psychological, Social, and Biological Foundations of Behavior	127	126◇128	75%	
MCAT Total	501	499◇503	54%	

Name: TOM JONES
Exam Date: 04/13/2015
AAMC ID: 20928474
Date of Birth: 01/07/1970

Notes

[1] Test scores, like other measurements, are not perfectly precise. The confidence bands around test scores mark the ranges in which the test taker's true scores probably lie. The diamond shapes and shading show that the test taker's true scores are more likely to be their reported scores (in the second column) than the other scores in the confidence bands.

[2] The percentile ranks of scores are the percentages of test takers who received the same scores or lower scores.

[3] For the four sections, non-overlapping confidence bands show a test taker's likely strengths and weaknesses. Overlapping confidence bands suggest that there are not meaningful differences in performance between sections.

the percentage of examinees who received the same score as you or a lower score. The ranks show your scores compared with the scores of other examinees.

Score Profiles

Score profiles are included to show your strengths and weaknesses across the four sections of the exam. This section of the score report can help you determine how to focus your preparation if you decide to retake the exam.

You can learn more about the score scale and score report at *aamc.org/students/applying/mcat/scores*.

Valid MCAT Scores

Each medical school sets its own policy about how much time can elapse between when you take the exam and when you apply, as well as the latest exam date it will accept during the application cycle. To find out the acceptable timing for the schools you're interested in, contact them directly or visit the Medical School Admission Requirements™ website, where there's a table showing which schools are accepting scores from the previous version of the MCAT exam in their admission cycles: *aamc.org/msar*.

Preparing for the Exam

While there's no one way to prepare for the MCAT exam, making sure you give yourself adequate time to prepare is critical. The amount of time you'll need to prepare really depends on you. Have you completed all the coursework that is associated with the content on the exam? Do you feel confident in all content areas? Are there some content topics or skills that you feel require more in-depth study or practice? Are you comfortable with the online testing format?

Students who take the MCAT exam and then complete the Post-MCAT Questionnaire report how much time they spent preparing for the exam (*aamc.org/data/pmq*). In recent years, the median amount of time students said they prepared was 20–21 hours per week for about three months. While there is no right or wrong way to prepare for the MCAT exam, you may find it useful to break down studying into manageable chunks, realizing that you can't tackle everything at once. This will also help give you a sense of the amount of time you'll need so you can prepare at a comfortable pace. The best study plans are those that you can tailor to your needs.

To help you develop your own study schedule:

- Get started by using this guide: *How to Create a Study Plan for the MCAT Exam* (*offers.aamc.org/mcat-study*).

- See how other examinees prepared with this collection of 21 testimonials: How I Prepared for the MCAT Exam (*students-residents.aamc.org/applying-medical-school/taking-mcat-exam/how-i-prepared-mcat-exam/*). Check out their study schedules, strategies, and the resources they used, and take note of their best advice about how to prepare.

To understand what's on the exam:

- Review this interactive content tool: **What's on the MCAT Exam?** (*students-residents.aamc.org/mcatexam*). It offers an overview of the exam sections, as well as details about the foundational concepts and skills you'll be asked to demonstrate on the exam. Each concept or skill has a link to a relevant Khan Academy MCAT Collection Tutorial.

- Read ***The Official Guide to the MCAT® Exam*** (*aamc.org/officialmcatguide*), which is the only official comprehensive overview of the exam. It includes 120 practice questions and solutions. The print book is available for purchase online at the AAMC Store and as an ebook through Amazon and Barnes & Noble.

- Visit *students-residents.aamc.org/mcatessentials* to read the ***MCAT® Essentials***.

To study the content on the exam:

- Visit **Khan Academy's MCAT Collection**. A series of video-based tutorials created to cover all the areas that the MCAT exam tests, the Khan Academy's MCAT collection was created in collaboration with the AAMC and the Robert Wood Johnson Foundation. Learn more at *khanacademy.org/test-prep/mcat*.

- Review the **Roadmap to MCAT Content in Sociology and Psychology Textbooks** (*students-residents.aamc.org/applying-medical-school/article/study-mcat-exam*). Publishers of introductory psychology and sociology textbooks have provided in the roadmap detailed information on where in their textbooks to find the concepts you'll need for the Psychological, Social, and Biological Foundations of Behavior section of the MCAT exam. Some of the textbooks in the roadmap are free, available online and in ebook format.

The AAMC has many official products, written by the test developers, to help you practice. There are full-length practice tests, as well as other resources that allow you to practice with large banks of questions. Learn more at *aamc.org/mcat/preparing*.

Test Dates, Registration, and Fees

In 2018, the MCAT exam will be administered 30 times from January through September. (The dates are posted on the MCAT website, *students-residents.aamc.org/mcatregister*.) Although the AAMC selects exam dates to ensure that scores are available to meet most medical school application deadlines, we recommend that you check the specific scheduling requirements of the schools of your choice, provided in the Medical School Admission Requirements website school profiles (*aamc.org/msar*).

To be sure that you get the most complete and up-to-date information about the MCAT exam, it is crucial that you read the *MCAT® Essentials* (available online at *students-residents.aamc.org/mcatessentials*) before you register for the exam. After you've read it, you can register online through the MCAT Registration System. There's a $315 fee for the exam, which covers both the cost of the test itself and the distribution of your scores. If you register late, make changes to your registration, and/or test at an international site, there are additional charges.

Many medical schools prefer that applicants take the MCAT exam in the spring rather than in the summer because of the short time between the availability of late-summer scores and school application deadlines, so consider taking the MCAT exam 12 to 18 months before your expected entry into medical school. However, it's important to remember that you should not take the exam before you feel ready. With limits in place for how often you can take the MCAT exam in a given year or over a lifetime (read the "Retaking the Exam" section of this chapter), you should have completed basic coursework and feel comfortable with your knowledge of introductory-level biology, general and organic chemistry, and physics—as well as first-semester psychology, sociology, and biochemistry—before you take it.

For more guidance on deciding when to take or retake the exam, please consult with your prehealth advisor.

Fee Assistance Program

The AAMC believes the cost of applying to medical school should not be a barrier to aspiring doctors. Therefore, the AAMC Fee Assistance Program helps qualifying examinees with MCAT registration fees, test preparation products, and other relevant AAMC products and services. To use the Fee Assistance Program, you must be approved for the benefit before registering for the exam. The benefits are not retroactive; you won't be given a refund for any resources or fees incurred before you qualify. Learn whether you're eligible for the Fee Assistance Program at *aamc.org/fap*.

Testing With Accommodations

The AAMC is committed to giving all individuals an opportunity to demonstrate their proficiency on the MCAT exam, and that includes ensuring access to people with disabilities in accordance with relevant law.

If you have a disability or medical condition that you believe requires an adjustment to the standard testing conditions, we encourage you to apply for accommodated testing.

For information about application timeframes and types of documentation needed, as well as how to apply, please see *aamc.org/mcat/accommodations*.

Retaking the Exam

It can be a tough decision, but if you're not happy with your performance on the MCAT exam, you have the option to take it again.

There are times when a retake is well worth considering. Perhaps you discovered that your coursework or study didn't cover the topics as thoroughly as you needed them to. Or there's a large discrepancy between your grade in a relevant subject and your score on a particular section. Or maybe you simply didn't feel well the day of the exam. In all these cases, prehealth advisors may be of great help, and we recommend you discuss the issue with yours. However, be aware that you can't choose which scores are sent to medical schools—admissions committees will see the results of all attempts at the exam that you choose to score. Additionally, there are limits on how often and how many times you may take the MCAT exam: You may take the exam up to three times in a testing year, up to four times in two consecutive years, and up to seven times in a lifetime. Voided exams and "no shows" count toward your attempts in a year or over your lifetime (however, these attempts are not included in the score report sent to medical schools).

Score Reporting

Your scores will be available in the MCAT Score Reporting System, accessible through the AAMC website at *apps.aamc.org/score-reporting-web*. No matter which option you use for sending your scores to medical schools, all attempts that are scored will be sent to them. You can't withhold any of your MCAT scores from your applications.

You have two options for sending your MCAT scores to medical schools:

- **Send your scores to the AMCAS® service:** The AMCAS service is the American Medical College Application Service®, which most U.S. medical schools take part in and which you will use to manage sending your application to participating institutions. Your MCAT scores are automatically released to AMCAS. This means that you don't need to take any additional steps to insert your scores into your application. You can view a list of participating schools at *aamc.org/amcas*. Read more about AMCAS in Chapter 7.

- **Send your scores to non-AMCAS schools:** If you're applying to non-AMCAS schools and programs, you'll need to send your scores electronically or by mailing a copy of your official score report to the non-AMCAS schools. Instructions are detailed in the MCAT Score Reporting System (*apps.aamc.org/ score-reporting-web*).

Gap Year and Career Changers: Taking the MCAT Exam

If you plan on taking a gap year(s) or are changing careers, you'll want to be thoughtful about preparing for the MCAT exam. Consider factors such as how well you know the content tested on the exam and when you would ideally want to begin medical school. This will help you figure out the best time to take the exam.

- **Know when you want to apply:** Many examinees consider taking their MCAT exam in the calendar year before the year they plan to enter medical school. For example, if you were applying in 2018 for entrance to medical school in 2019, you would take the exam in 2018. If you plan on taking a gap year(s), think about whether you want to take the exam before, during, or after that time, and build in time to prepare.

- **Mastering the content:** You are the best judge of how prepared you are. First, determine whether there's coursework you need to take or whether you need more time to study. Some applicants also need to take additional coursework, retake coursework that is several years old, or complete postbaccalaureate programs in order to meet application requirements. Consider this when choosing an exam date because the timeline may affect whether the exam will still be accepted by various medical schools.

- **Retesting and testing limits:** If you think you might need to test more than once in a calendar year, try to schedule an exam date early in the year. This will give you more time to receive your scores and prepare for a retest. Remember: You can take the exam only three times in a single testing year, four times over two consecutive testing years, and seven times in a lifetime.

If you've never taken the MCAT exam and you don't currently have a prehealth advisor to help you prepare, the **National Association of Advisors for the Health Professions** has volunteer advisors available. More information is at *naahp.org*.

> **Worksheets at the end of chapters in this guide are available in fillable PDF format at *aamc.org/msar-resources*.**

Ask yourself these questions when you're getting ready for the MCAT exam.

- Am I familiar with what will be on the exam?   ❏ Yes   ❏ No   ❏ Unsure
  (Find out what's on the exam: *students-residents.aamc.org/mcatexam*.)

- If no or unsure, what content or sections am I unsure about? _____

- Have I allowed enough time to study and feel comfortable with my knowledge of the content
  on the exam?

     o Chemical and Physical Foundations of Biological Systems

          ❏ Yes   ❏ No, I need more time   ❏ Unsure

     o Biological and Biochemical Foundations of Living Systems

          ❏ Yes   ❏ No, I need more time   ❏ Unsure

     o Psychological, Social, and Biological Foundations of Behavior

          ❏ Yes   ❏ No, I need more time   ❏ Unsure

     o Critical Analysis and Reasoning Skills

          ❏ Yes   ❏ No, I need more time   ❏ Unsure

If you have areas where you need more study, check out the AAMC's preparation resources, which offer
the opportunity to get familiar with the online testing environment. Also, consider forming a study group
at your school or with other applicants who are preparing for the exam. Talk to your prehealth advisor
about resources you may have on campus or through your institution.

- Am I within one to two calendar years of wanting to apply to medical school?

          ❏ Yes   ❏ No   ❏ Unsure

- Have I spoken with my prehealth advisor? Does my advisor agree that I am ready?

          ❏ Yes   ❏ No   ❏ Unsure

- Have I applied to see if I qualify for the Fee Assistance Program?

          ❏ Yes   ❏ No   ❏ Unsure

- Do I feel prepared and ready to take the exam?

          ❏ Yes   ❏ No   ❏ Unsure

If you answered "no" to many of these questions, consult with your prehealth advisor about developing a
plan to take the exam. See *aamc.org/mcat* for information about creating a study plan. When you're close
to registering for a test date, be sure to read the *MCAT® Essentials* for important information on scheduling,
registration, test day policies, and scoring (*students-residents.aamc.org/mcatessentials*).

CHAPTER 6

Choosing Your Schools

Applying to medical school can be both exciting and stressful. For me, one of the more exciting parts was that I had a choice about where I applied. There were three key things that I looked at when I was exploring my medical school options. First, I met with current medical students to get to hear their perspective of the medical school. Second, I read through each school's website and their mission statement. Third, I looked at the location.

Hearing about students' experiences from medical schools I was interested in gave me a lot of perspective and insight about the culture, curriculum, student life, and values of the institution. I was also keenly aware of the deficit of doctors in my home state, and I wanted to attend a medical school that sought to ameliorate this problem. I specifically looked to see if that was included in the school's mission statement. Finally, I'm a homebody; I like my home state and love being close to family. My school is about 45 minutes from where I grew up. It's close to my family, church, and friends.

You may think that you need to apply to a long list of schools, but doing your research can help you narrow your choices down to the schools that are the best fit. Look at mission statements but don't neglect meeting with current students to hear about their experiences there. And don't forget to look within yourself. Your values, needs, and choices are a key factor in deciding where to apply and where to attend.

Weston Eldridge
MD Candidate
University of Mississippi
School of Medicine
Class of 2021

The Overall Mission of the School

Many of the differences among medical schools are obvious. Some schools are located on the East Coast, some on the West. Some are private; others, public. Some have a large entering class; others, small. Some have multiple campuses by way of regional campuses. And, as explained in Chapter 3, medical schools vary in the content of their courses, in the way they teach, and even in the way they grade and evaluate students.

These are all factors you'll want to consider as you narrow your selection, and we touch on them in the following pages. But the differences go even deeper, and at a very core level, medical schools have diverse missions and priorities. Because of these distinctions, what is significant to one school may be of only moderate importance to another, and these qualities naturally carry into the selection process.

Deciding where to apply requires that you become aware of the differences among schools, which is crucial, but it's also important to analyze yourself—your skills, experiences, career goals, and so forth—to identify the most appropriate matches. Take, for instance, an institution that places a strong emphasis on primary care. Is that the career path you intend to follow? If so, and especially if you can demonstrate your interest through extensive experience related to that area, you become a more attractive candidate on that basis alone.

That's one example. Other schools may be actively seeking students from specific geographic or rural areas. Others may be looking for students with a high potential for a research career. Still others may want to increase the number of doctors who plan to practice in their state (often a goal of public institutions). The differing missions among schools are reflected in their admission policies and standards.

If you need help with this self-analysis, think back to the various experiences you've had over the years. The ones you found especially rewarding or inspirational are likely to correlate with a specific area of interest and, by extension, a career goal.

Did you volunteer for two summers at a clinic in a **rural, underserved area**? Perhaps that's the direction you'd like to take your career in. If so, you'll want to seek out medical schools that place a high priority in that area.

Were the part-time jobs you had while doing research particularly gratifying? If you'd like to pursue a **research career**, look for schools that have a strong reputation in that area or are known for graduating a large percentage of medical students pursuing research careers.

Your interests and career goals are also demonstrated in other ways. Did you spend your junior year tutoring freshmen and sophomores in entry-level biology or chemistry? Perhaps you'd like to join a **medical school faculty** and educate the next generation of physicians. If so, find medical schools that have a relatively large percentage of graduates in teaching positions, and check whether the schools are affiliated with teaching hospitals.

Once again, keep in mind that applying to medical school is a two-way street. While you're looking for a match, so are the schools. Your experiences will provide good insights for the admissions officers and help them determine whether your interests and their missions are congruent. If you don't know which medical career path you want to pursue yet, that's okay. Aim to get as many rich and diverse experiences as possible so you will be a well-rounded applicant.

Kicking Off Your Research

There are several ways you can research schools to identify the ones that best match your own strengths, interests, and goals. Here are some factors to consider in making your selection:

- Research reputation and opportunities
- Community-based experiences and opportunities
- Geographic location
- School's teaching methods
- Program of elective courses
- Faculty mentorship
- Placement of recent graduates in specialty residencies
- Residency programs at hospitals affiliated with the school

The Medical School Admission Requirements™ website: Start your research with the medical school profiles on this site, *aamc.org/msar*. Here, each institution includes a clear mission statement and a description of its selection factors.

School websites and literature: You'll also want to review information provided by schools themselves. Although the specific content varies by school, each includes detailed material for prospective students.

Advisors: Your prehealth advisor or career counselor will be able to recommend specific schools likely to be a good "fit." These advisors have a lot of insight about the application process, so don't overlook this resource. Also, make sure you attend health career fairs to speak with admissions staff from medical schools and participate in premed or prehealth student organizations.

The Educational Program

It's easy to get caught up in a specific region or location, or you may recognize the name of a prestigious school and want to go there simply because it sounds impressive. You'll want to consider all your options, though. As you weigh your decision, you'll also want to consider the differences among the educational programs themselves.

There's likely going to be a strong relationship between a school's mission and its **curriculum**. You'll be able to gauge whether an institution's objectives align with your interests by analyzing course requirements and elective programs. A medical school with a mission to graduate more primary care doctors may, for example, have a track that provides additional training in that area. A school that emphasizes research may require their students to write a thesis or devote an extended period of time to scholarly pursuits.

As you do your research, also consider what **teaching methods** you find most effective. Do you tend to do well with self-directed or participatory learning exercises, or do you prefer a learning environment with the more traditional, lecture-based style? Although most medical schools use an educational model that combines a variety of methods, every program adapts their own design. Are you looking for classes that promote small-group discussions and problem-based learning exercises? Or are you more comfortable with a traditional teaching approach? Eventually, these are great topics to discuss with current students, but a good starting point for your exploration is a school's website, as well as the AAMC's curriculum directory (*aamc.org/initiatives/cir*).

There are many other factors you might want to think about. How will you be evaluated? At what point must students pass the first two steps of the United States Medical Licensing Examination (USMLE) before advancing in their education? What level of academic support is available? Is there a mentor system, for instance? What about cultural organizations and support services for minority and first-generation students—are they available? Questions such as these will undoubtedly enter into your final decision making.

How Do GPA and MCAT Scores Factor In?

Don't choose schools based solely on where you think your grades and MCAT® scores will be accepted. While there's no question that your educational record is important and that admissions officers seek candidates who are likely to succeed academically in their programs, it's important to realize that academics alone do not predict who will become an effective physician, and admissions officers know that all too well.

The fact that there are many instances in which a "high-scoring" applicant is not accepted to a medical school—and in which an applicant with lower-than-average grades and scores is—tells you that admissions officers must be looking at other factors.

Admissions officers are taking a more holistic approach to evaluating applicants. Through this practice, admissions officers assess candidates more broadly, looking not only at their "metrics" (GPA and MCAT scores) but also at their experiences and personal attributes.

You can read about the holistic approach to admissions in Chapter 8, "The Admission Decision."

Attending Medical School in Your Home State

State residents enrolled in state-supported medical schools pay lower tuition than nonresidents. In addition, in-state residents are often given preference for admission (compared with out-of-state residents) for at least some of their spaces because the school receives state government support. With this in mind, you may want to give strong consideration to the public institutions in your state as you decide where to apply. Note that residency requirements are established by each state. Check with individual medical schools for policies regarding qualifying for in-state or residential status.

Nationally, 61% of 2017 matriculants attended schools in their home states.

International Students

There's only a small number of international students—those who are not U.S. citizens or permitted to reside permanently in this country—at U.S. medical schools. If you are an international applicant, know that private medical schools are more likely to accept international students than public schools, and that most medical schools require completion of premedical coursework at a U.S. college or university. For more information, see the Aspiring Docs® fact sheet on applying as an international applicant at *aamc.org/aspiringdocs*.

Public or Private?

You may also be deliberating between public and private institutions. Typically, the most cost-effective option is to consider a public medical school in the state where you live. (If you're from out of state, the cost differential between a public and a private school virtually disappears. See Table 10.1 in Chapter 10.) But don't automatically assume, even if you're interested in a state school near your home, that the private route will be more expensive under all circumstances. Some private institutions have large endowments that allow them to provide significant scholarship aid to qualifying students. These scholarships lower the "effective" tuition rate and permit those students to graduate with less educational debt than they would have if they had attended a public medical school in their home state.

Cost is only one consideration, though. Another element to be aware of when investigating the differences between private and public institutions is the school's mission—and how it might relate to your own aspirations and interests. Although all medical schools—public or private—have different missions, certain public institutions may have specific goals related to their state, such as increasing the supply of physicians. (If the school is in your home state and you'd like to live and work there after graduation, that will be a factor from both your perspective and the school's.) Other public institutions were founded by state legislators with an emphasis on the needs of a particular patient population—such as elderly, rural, or underserved groups— which should enter into your evaluation if that objective corresponds to your own career intentions.

Additional Factors to Consider

There are many other factors that may be important to you as you search for a good "fit," including these:

Location. Perhaps you simply prefer a specific geographic region. Do you want to be close to family and friends? Do you prefer a warmer (or cooler) climate? Are you a fan of the East Coast … or the South … or the West? What about a bustling city environment versus a rural one? These factors play to your comfort level, and all are valid considerations. Beyond that, though, location can also relate to your career goals, as well as to a school's mission. If you hope to specialize in geriatrics, for example, a medical school located in an area with a higher-than-average proportion of older adults may be your best choice.

That's looking at it from your perspective. Consider, for a moment, the school's perspective. In some cases, a school may be seeking students from particular geographic regions in order to bolster its diversity, and you'll want to consider the impact—if any—that your own state residence might have on your application to medical schools in other areas. On the other hand, there are schools that look for local, in-state students who will continue to work and contribute to communities in that state. Review each school's mission statement to see what they're seeking in their applicants.

Size and Demographics. The size and demographics of the medical school—both in terms of its student body and its faculty—may be a consideration for you as well. The school entries in the Medical School Admission Requirements website contain data on the prior year's entering class, including the number of students by gender as well as by self-reported identification (*aamc.org/msar*).

Costs. Medical education is expensive, and the expenses associated with particular institutions will no doubt be a factor in your decision. You won't know what your actual costs will be (or the degree of assistance you will receive) until a school sends you a financial aid package in conjunction with its acceptance offer. Still, in looking through the school entries in the Medical School Admission Requirements website, you can get a general idea about the relative expenses of each institution, and you can take those numbers into consideration as you narrow your selection.

"Additional" doesn't mean less important. Figure 6.1 shows what matriculating students felt about specific factors in deciding which school to attend.

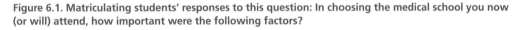

Figure 6.1. Matriculating students' responses to this question: In choosing the medical school you now (or will) attend, how important were the following factors?

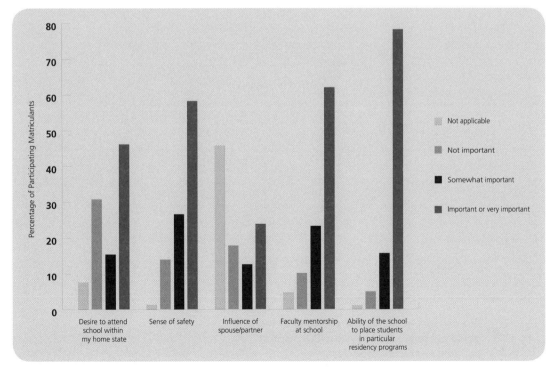

Source: AAMC's 2017 Matriculating Student Questionnaire (MSQ).

Special Regional Opportunities

Finally, you should be aware that some states without a public medical school participate in special interstate and regional agreements that give their residents access to a medical education. Currently, there are five interstate agreements:

- The Delaware Institute of Medical Information and Research

  dhss.delaware.gov/dhss/dhcc/dimer.html
  1-302-577-3240
  1-800-292-7935

- The Finance Authority of Maine's Access to Medical Education Program

  famemaine.com/fi
  1-800-228-3734

- University of Utah School of Medicine Idaho Contract

  medicine.utah.edu/students/programs/md/admissions/residency-non-residency.php
  1-801-581-7498

- The Western Interstate Commission for Higher Education

  wiche.edu/psep/medi
  1-303-541-0200

- The WWAMI (Washington, Wyoming, Alaska, Montana, and Idaho) Program

  uwmedicine.washington.edu/Education/WWAMI/Pages/Medical-School.aspx

You can learn more about each of these regional opportunities by visiting their websites or calling their program offices.

> **Worksheets at the end of chapters in this guide are available in fillable PDF format at *aamc.org/msar-resources*.**

Use this form to identify and assess the schools where you may apply.

The Medical School Admission Requirement website allows you to filter your search for different medical schools by things such as class size, location, and community service requirement (*aamc.org/msar*). Every medical school has a different curriculum and style. This worksheet can help you determine which factors are important to you.

School name: _____

Factor	Ideal fit	Good fit	No opinion	Unsure	Not a fit	Notes
Course offerings						
Class size						
Location						
Research programs						
Technology						
Interviews and/or meetings with faculty						
Reputation						
Technology						
Tuition and financial aid						
Programs for minority or disadvantaged students						
Teaching methods						
Combined-degree offerings						
Campus tour						
Rural or community offerings						
Residency placement						

Impression of school: ❏ Favorable   ❏ Undecided   ❏ Unfavorable

Likelihood of applying: ❏ Will apply   ❏ Undecided   ❏ Unlikely to apply

Follow-up questions to ask: _____

CHAPTER 7

Applying to Medical School

> My AMCAS application started out as purple ink on a piece of scrap paper on a tired train ride home to Brooklyn. During that hour-long ride, I covered that paper with fragments of patient encounters, personal experiences, and lessons learned. I love that the beginning of such a formal process was s o spontaneous, because it led to the most honest of thoughts.
>
> As that purple ink became black typeface on a computer screen, I worked extensively for many months both on my own and with advisors so that there was a clear, coherent, and concise narrative that was still true to the honesty of those initial thoughts and feelings from that train ride. That's often the most difficult part of the writing process: making sure that beneath the formal language and after the countless revisions, your application still sounds like you. This is crucial in helping others understand your narrative and your reasons for pursuing medicine. For me, the best way to do this was to start the writing process early, share my work with people who are familiar with the medical school application process, and continuously ask myself if my writing was true to my experience.
>
> It's impossible to do this perfectly, but what's important is that you put significant thought into getting as close as you can. Ultimately, I think that this commitment to your voice is one of the most important things in putting you in the best position for not only a smooth application process but also a fulfilling career.

Slavena Salve Nissan
MD Candidate
Icahn School of Medicine at Mount Sinai
Class of 2020

Responsibilities of the Medical School Applicant

As a medical school applicant, you have certain responsibilities. These are reviewed at length at the end of this chapter, but some of the most critical are:

- Meeting all deadlines
- Completing the AMCAS® application accurately
- Knowing the admission requirements at each school
- Promptly updating your AMCAS application with any change in contact information
- Responding promptly to interview invitations
- Filing for financial aid as soon as possible
- Withdrawing from the schools you will not attend

For more details, read "AAMC's Application and Acceptance Protocols for Applicants and Admissions Officers" later in this chapter.

American Medical College Application Service®

You may have heard about the American Medical College Application Service (AMCAS®) from your prehealth advisor, career counselor, or even your classmates. AMCAS is a centralized medical school application processing service offered by the AAMC and used by almost every medical school in the country. This service does not screen applicants; rather, it provides admissions officers with the information and tools they need to select the applicants who are the best fit for their institution.

AMCAS offers many benefits to applicants. The most obvious one is that it allows you to apply to as many medical schools as you want with a single application (although many schools require a secondary application, a topic discussed later in this chapter). It also provides applicants with a single point of transmission for official transcripts, letters of evaluation, and other supporting documentation.

Even if you're not yet ready to begin the application process, you can familiarize yourself with it at *aamc.org/amcas*. There, you'll find an application overview, tips for completing an application, frequently asked questions, video tutorials, and the comprehensive *AMCAS® Applicant Guide*.

If you have previously registered for the MCAT® exam, the Fee Assistance Program, or other AAMC programs and services, you've already created an AAMC username and password and received an AAMC ID. Use this same information to access the AMCAS application site. If you don't already have an AAMC ID number, you'll need to register online to create a username and password before you begin your application.

AMCAS Application Sections

The AMCAS application has nine sections. That may sound like a lot, but remember, you don't have to complete it all at once. You can save your work and return to your application as many times as you want until you finish and are ready to submit it. Here's an overview of what to expect:

1. **Identifying Information.** This section asks you to enter your name, birth information, and gender identity or expression.

2. **Schools Attended.** Here, you'll enter high school and college information. Once you've completed this section (and the identifying information section), you'll be able to create a Transcript Request Form, which will help you request official transcripts from your registrar.

3. **Biographic Information.** You'll use this section to enter your contact information, citizenship status, legal residence, ethnicity, language(s) spoken, and other biographic information. Also, you'll indicate your immigration status in the Citizenship subsection. If the U.S. government approved your Deferred Action for Childhood Arrivals (DACA) application, you may select "DACA" from the designated drop-down list.

4. **Coursework.** You'll enter grades and credits for every course you've enrolled in at any U.S., U.S. territorial, or Canadian postsecondary institution that appears on your official college transcript(s). You're required to provide information for all the college-level courses you've taken, even if you took them during high school. For courses attempted through a study abroad program, carefully follow the instructions outlined in the *AMCAS® Applicant Guide*. List study-abroad coursework under the foreign college, the foreign listing of your home institution, or the organization at which it was attempted. Do not enter the coursework twice.

5. **Work/Activities.** Here, you'll enter any work and extracurricular activities, awards, honors, or publications that you'd like to bring to the attention of the medical schools. You may list up to 15 experiences. You'll then choose the three you consider to be the most meaningful and have up to 1,325 characters to explain why each experience was particularly meaningful to you.

6. **Letters of Evaluation.** In this section, you'll provide information about people writing letters of evaluation on your behalf. You may want to review the AAMC's Letters of Evaluation Guidelines, a useful tool developed to help your letter writers. (This step is covered in more detail later in the chapter.)

7. **Medical Schools.** In this section, you'll designate the medical schools to which you want to submit an application. In addition, you can designate which letters of evaluation you wish to send to specific schools.

8. **Personal Statement.** Here, you'll compose an essay about why you want to go to medical school. (This is discussed more thoroughly later in this chapter.)

9. **Standardized Tests.** And finally … your MCAT scores. In this section, you'll review your MCAT scores and enter any additional test information, such as GRE scores. Any MCAT scores from 2003 or later will automatically be released to AMCAS. Please note: It's important to include all the MCAT exams you're scheduled to take on your AMCAS application and update this information as appropriate after you submit your application.

This is a simplified overview of the AMCAS application. Read the *AMCAS® Applicant Guide* and explore the various resources for a more thorough understanding of the application on the AMCAS website at *aamc.org/amcas*.

Transcript Requests via AMCAS

In addition to completing your AMCAS application, you must request that official transcripts from all postsecondary institutions at which you've registered be sent to AMCAS. AMCAS provides a Transcript Request Form to facilitate this process with your registrar(s). If you've taken courses at a junior college, community college, trade school, or other professional school—regardless of whether you earned credit—within the United States, Canada, or U.S. territories, you must provide an official transcript from that institution. (This requirement also applies to any college courses you took in high school.) For most applicants, all official transcripts must be received no later than two weeks after the deadline date for application materials. Please refer to the *AMCAS® Applicant Guide* at *aamc.org/amcasguide* and the AMCAS website for detailed information about official transcript requirements.

Limited Changes After Submission

It's important to check your work carefully before you hit "submit" because you're limited in what changes you can make after submission. You can make changes to your contact information (such as addresses and emails) and add schools or letters of evaluation, but other than that, your application will be submitted to schools exactly as it was completed.

Application Processing and Verification

Once AMCAS has received your submitted application and all required official transcripts from each postsecondary school where you were registered, the AMCAS verification process begins. AMCAS verifies the accuracy of your academic record by comparing the information you entered on your application with what's on your official transcripts. During the verification process, AMCAS converts transcript grades to AMCAS grades based on conversion information provided by colleges and universities and calculates an AMCAS GPA. The AMCAS GPA gives medical schools a standard way to compare each applicant's academic record. AMCAS GPAs may differ from the GPA shown on your records at the institutions you attended.

Once verification is complete, AMCAS makes your application and MCAT scores available to all the medical schools you designated (MCAT scores from 2003 and later are automatically included).

The Application and Admission Cycle

The AMCAS application usually opens to applicants in early May of each year and opens for submission in early June. Participating schools receive verified application data from AMCAS in late June.

The deadlines for receipt of primary applications to medical schools that participate in AMCAS are from the Early Decision Deadline in early August to mid-December (information on secondary applications is discussed later in this chapter). However, there's no single application timetable because each school establishes its own deadlines for receipt of required materials. You can find specific dates on medical schools' websites and in the school listings on the Medical School Admission Requirements™ website (*aamc.org/msar*).

Medical schools vary in the timing of their admission decisions. Most schools use a system of "rolling admissions," selecting students for interviews and making admission decisions as applications are received, rather than waiting until after a specific deadline date to begin their evaluation process. All medical schools must wait until mid-October to start offering acceptance letters. You can find out if a medical school uses a rolling admissions system by checking its website.

For the 2017 AMCAS application cycle, students applied to 16 schools, on average. The U.S. medical schools that are not participating in AMCAS for the 2018 entering class are mostly in Texas. The seven public medical schools in Texas listed below participate in the Texas Medical and Dental School Application Service (TMDSAS) for those pursuing the MD degree. You can learn more about this application service and apply to these schools through TMDSAS at *utsystem.edu/tmdsas*. Applicants pursuing MD-PhD degrees at all but the Paul L. Foster School of Medicine can do so through AMCAS, however.

If you're interested in schools that do not participate in AMCAS, please contact them directly for application instructions.

- Sophie Davis Biomedical Education Program/CUNY School of Medicine

- McGovern Medical School at the University of Texas Health Science Center at Houston

- Texas A&M Health Science Center College of Medicine

- Texas Tech University Health Sciences Center School of Medicine

- Texas Tech University Health Sciences Center Paul L. Foster School of Medicine

- University of Texas Southwestern Medical School

- University of Texas Medical Branch School of Medicine

- University of Texas Health Science Center at San Antonio Long School of Medicine

You should also contact schools directly for application information if you wish to pursue a joint degree program, such as a baccalaureate-MD or an MD-PhD.

As far as interviews go, many admissions committees begin meeting with candidates in the late summer and continue through spring. However, most interviews are held during the winter months. (This part of the admission cycle is discussed in Chapter 8.) By March 30, medical schools will have issued enough acceptances to at least equal the size of their first-year entering class.

Personal Statements and Letters of Evaluation

As you'll learn in Chapter 8, "The Admission Decision," admissions officers want to know more about you than just where you went to college, the courses you've taken, the grades you've earned, and how you scored on the MCAT exam. They want to know you on a more personal level. That's why an essay and letters of evaluation are integral components of your medical school application.

Your Personal Statement

Every applicant is required to submit a personal essay of up to 5,300 characters (about one page) in length. This is your opportunity to distinguish yourself from other applicants and provide admissions officers with insights about why you're interested in medicine—and why you would be a dedicated and effective physician.

Most admissions committees place significant weight on this section, so take the time to craft an organized, well-written, and compelling statement. Here are some questions you may want to consider while writing your essay:

- Why do you want a career in medicine?

- What motivates you to learn more about medicine?

- What should medical schools know about you that isn't described in other sections of the application?

In addition, you may wish to include information such as this:

- What hardships, challenges, or obstacles have influenced your educational pursuits?

- Are you able to explain significant fluctuations in your academic record not explained elsewhere in your application?

It's a good idea to use specific examples in your essay. Instead of writing "Challenges in my childhood led me to consider medicine at an early age," write, "The summer I turned 8, my 11-year-old sister was diagnosed with neuroblastoma, and I witnessed firsthand the compassion and understanding with which the doctor dealt with my parents. It was during those first few difficult months that I decided I wanted to be a physician."

Additionally, ensure that your essay is interesting, follows a logical and orderly flow, and relates to your reasons for choosing medicine and/or why you believe you'll be successful in medical school and as a physician. Beyond that, be sure to use correct grammar and avoid typographical errors and misspellings.

For MD-PhD Applicants

If you're applying to MD-PhD programs, you'll be required to write two additional essays: a relatively brief one focusing on your reasons for pursuing the combined degree and a lengthier one (about three pages) describing your research activities. You can read more about these additional essays in the *2018 AMCAS®* *Applicant Guide* or get further guidance from your prehealth advisor or career counselor.

Early Decision Programs

One of your first decisions will be whether to apply to a medical school through the Early Decision Program (EDP) or the regular application process. Although criteria for accepting EDP applicants vary among schools, programs frequently require that applicants show extraordinary credentials. A small percentage of applicants apply through the EDP, and only about half of medical schools offer the option. You can learn more about program requirements at *aamc.org/students/applying*.

Letters of Evaluation

In the Letters of Evaluation section, you'll provide information about the people writing your letters. Although you can add up to 10 letter entries, medical schools do not necessarily wish to receive 10 letters per applicant. Most schools request only two or three letters. (You can find the minimum and maximum letters accepted by each school on the Medical School Admission Requirements website.) AMCAS accepts letters of evaluation on behalf of participating medical schools. This service enables medical schools to receive all letters electronically from AMCAS and allows letter writers to send their letter to AMCAS, rather than to each individual school. AMCAS permits additional letters so that you have the option to designate specific letters for specific schools. For more information and a current list of schools participating in the AMCAS Letter Service, see *aamc.org/aboutamcasletters*.

Medical schools have various requirements for letters of evaluation, but they all require letters in one form or another. If your college has a prehealth advisor, medical schools will probably require a letter from this individual (or from the prehealth committee, if your school has one), as well as a letter from at least one faculty member. In instances where there is no prehealth advisor, many medical schools may ask for additional letters from faculty and often specify that at least one comes from a science professor.

Some medical schools don't specify who should write your letters and welcome additional letters beyond the required ones. However, be aware of any limits on the number they will accept. In all cases, you should review medical schools' websites or the Medical School Admission Requirements website for information on specific letter requirements (*aamc.org/msar*).

Medical schools want letters from people who are in a position to judge your ability to be successful in medical school, which includes not only your academic capabilities and accomplishments, but also your personal characteristics and skills.

Secondary Applications

Your primary application is your AMCAS application, and it provides admissions officers with much of the information they need. However, most medical schools also require a school-specific, or "secondary," application because it allows them to assess students' reasons for applying to that particular school. (Medical schools will notify you if they would like you to fill out a secondary application, although you can also find out by looking at their profiles on the Medical School Admission Requirements website.) Secondary applications may call for additional letters of evaluation, supplemental writing samples, and updated transcripts. Go to the websites of the medical schools you're interested in to learn more.

Application Fees

Medical school application fees fall into four general categories:

- *AMCAS Application.* For the 2018 application cycle, the AMCAS application fee plus designation to one school was $160, and it cost $39 for each additional school. Check the AMCAS website for the latest application fee information. Remember, some schools don't use AMCAS, and you may pay different fees in those instances.

- *Secondary Application.* In 2017, fees for secondary applications ranged from $0 to $200.

- *College Service Fees.* Your college registrar may charge a small fee to send your transcript to AMCAS. Occasionally, you'll incur a fee to send your letters of evaluation to AMCAS.

- *MCAT Exam Fees.* Although technically not part of the application fee, the costs associated with the MCAT exam are a necessary component of the overall process. The initial registration fee for the MCAT exam is currently $310 and covers the cost of the exam and distribution of your scores. In addition, you may incur fees for late registration, changes to your registration, or testing at international test sites.

You can read more about the MCAT exam in Chapter 5 and get up-to-date information on the MCAT website (*aamc.org/mcat*).

For more information on application fees, go to *aamc.org/first/factsheets*.

Criminal Background Check

The AAMC facilitates a national background check on all accepted applicants to participating medical schools via Certiphi Screening, Inc. This service provides required background checks to medical schools and prevents you from paying additional fees to each medical school to run these checks independently. For more information, go to *aamc.org/amcascbc*.

Be aware that participating medical schools may also require applicants to undergo a separate national background check process, if it's required by their own institutional regulations or by applicable state law.

Fee Assistance Program

The AAMC believes that the cost of applying to medical school should not be a financial barrier to people interested in becoming physicians.

The AAMC Fee Assistance Program helps MCAT examinees and AMCAS applicants who, without financial assistance, would be unable to take the MCAT exam and apply to medical schools that use the AMCAS application. Visit the Fee Assistance Program website at *aamc.org/fap* for details about the program's eligibility requirements and to access the application. You'll be able to use your Fee Assistance Program award benefits for up to two calendar years. Benefits expire on December 31 the year after they are awarded, regardless of when in the year you apply for, and receive, the award. **You may only apply for fee assistance once per calendar year. Fee Assistance Program benefits are never retroactive**.

Applicants who are approved for fee assistance in 2018 will receive MCAT, AMCAS, and Medical School Admission Requirements benefits.

MCAT Benefits

- Reduced registration fees for up to four MCAT exam dates

- Reduced rescheduling fees for MCAT exam dates

- A suite of MCAT prep products and resources (you'll receive more details about these benefits if you're awarded fee assistance)

- Up to $800 toward an updated psychoeducational or medical evaluation if it's required to support your MCAT accommodations application

Regardless of how many times you're awarded fee assistance, you'll receive MCAT prep product benefits only once.

Medical School Admission Requirements Benefits

- Complimentary access to the MSAR® website until December 31, 2018 ($56 value)

AMCAS Benefits

- Waiver for all AMCAS fees for one application submission with up to 16 medical school designations ($730 value)

Additional fees will be charged for each medical school designation beyond the initial set of 16.

Special Note About Deferred Entry

In recent years, most medical schools have developed delayed-matriculation policies to allow accepted applicants to defer entry without giving up their spot. Deferrals are granted only after acceptance. These programs usually require that you submit a written request, and some schools also ask for a report at the end of the deferral period. Matriculation delays are usually granted for one year, although some schools occasionally defer for longer periods of time. Some institutions may require delayed matriculants to sign an agreement not to apply to other medical schools in the interim, while others permit applications to other schools. If you're interested in this option, you should seek specific information from schools you applied to. You can find out more about each school's policy by viewing their profile on the Medical School Admission Requirements website.

Gap Year and Career Changers

If you're applying to medical school after spending more than a year out of college, you'll need to get transcripts from any additional coursework or degree programs you've completed since your undergraduate graduation. Even if you applied previously to medical school, you'll need to resubmit official transcripts. Also, you must resubmit letters of evaluation to AMCAS each time you apply.

For more information about gap years, please look for the "Making the Most of Your Gap Year" fact sheet online at *students-residents.aamc.org/applying-medical-school/article/making-most-your-gap-year*.

AAMC's Application and Acceptance Protocols for Applicants and Admissions Officers

The AAMC recommends certain protocols, outlined in the following boxes, to help ensure that all MD and MD-PhD applicants receive timely notification about the outcome of their application and protect schools and programs from having unfilled positions in their entering classes. Admissions officers and prehealth advisors often refer to these protocols as "traffic rules." Prospective applicants, their advisors, and admissions staff at medical schools and programs should all be aware of these application and acceptance protocols for applicants.

What This Means for You (the Applicant)

These protocols were developed to ensure fairness for both applicants and medical schools. By reading and acknowledging the guidelines, as well as agreeing to adhere to them, applicants and medical schools affirm that they understand the timelines and stresses involved with making these important decisions. They also acknowledge that their decisions affect the choices of other applicants and schools that are also in the midst of making acceptance and admission decisions. Admissions officers know that most applicants are anxiously awaiting notifications, but their committees are also diligently working to build the next class for their medical schools. These rules help ensure that everyone does their best to make timely, ethical, and fair decisions during this hectic time. The protocols are periodically reviewed by the AAMC's Committee on Admission and approved by the AAMC's Council of Deans. The following protocols were approved May 7, 2018.

Application and Acceptance Protocols for Applicants

The AAMC recommends the following steps to help ensure that all MD and MD-PhD applicants receive timely notification about the outcome of their applications and to protect schools and programs from having unfilled positions in their entering classes. These protocols are often referred to as "Traffic Rules" by admissions officers and prehealth advisors. Prospective applicants, their advisors, and admissions staff at medical schools and programs should all be aware of these Application and Acceptance Protocols for applicants. An applicant's actions during the admissions process should be conducted in the spirit of professionalism and ethics expected of a future physician.

These guidelines are not intended to supersede the policies, timelines, or discretion of individual schools or programs. Each applicant is expected to become familiar with the procedures and requirements of each school to which they apply. The AAMC understands that an individual's circumstances (e.g., delays in receiving financial aid offer or other compelling personal reasons) may warrant exception from one or more of the following protocols and defers to each school's judgment in such cases. Below are AAMC recommendations for applicants to an MD or MD-PhD program:

1. Understand and comply with these Applicant Responsibilities as well as with the application, acceptance, and admission procedures at each school or program to which you apply.

2. Provide accurate and truthful information in all aspects of your application, interview(s), acceptance, and admission processes for each school or program to which you apply.

3. Submit all application documents (e.g., primary and secondary application forms, transcript[s], letters of evaluation/recommendation, fees, etc.) on or before the school or program's published deadline date.

4. Notify all relevant medical school application services of any change, permanent or temporary, to your contact information (e.g., mailing address, telephone number, and email address).

5. If you will be unavailable for an extended period of time (e.g., during foreign travel, vacation, holidays) during the application/admission process:

    a. Provide instructions regarding your application, and if applicable, delegate the authority to respond to any offers of acceptance to a parent or other responsible individual in your absence.
    b. Inform all schools or programs at which your application remains under consideration of this person's name, contact information, and authority to act on your behalf. Include dates of your unavailability and inclusive dates for the designation of authority to act on your behalf.

6. Respond promptly to a school's or program's invitation for an interview. If you cannot appear for a previously scheduled interview, notify the school or program **immediately** that you need to cancel.

7. Begin promptly the steps necessary to determine your eligibility for financial aid. This may include filing need-analysis forms early and encouraging your parents (when required) to file the appropriate income tax forms.

8. In fairness to other applicants, if you have decided before April 30 not to attend a medical school or program that has offered you an acceptance, **promptly** withdraw your application from that school(s) or program(s).

9. Out of respect for other applicants, if you receive an offer of acceptance from more than one school or program:

    (a) Withdraw your acceptance from any school or program you do not plan to attend as soon as you have made that decision;
    (b) On or before April 15, narrow your selection(s) to no more than three schools or programs and withdraw your acceptance(s) from all other schools or programs; and
    (c) On or before April 30, choose the school or program to which you plan to matriculate and promptly withdraw your acceptances from all other schools or programs.

10. If you receive additional acceptances following April 30, it is your responsibility to promptly notify any school(s) you have decided to not attend. Your decision should be made by the deadline established by the medical school(s).

11. To the extent you have not already done so in furtherance of paragraphs 9 and 10 above, withdraw your acceptance(s) from all other schools or programs as soon as you matriculate at a U.S. or Canadian school or program. For the purposes of these protocols, *matriculation* means that a student has begun a pre-matriculation program, attended orientation immediately preceding enrollment, or enrolled in classes at a medical school.

Approved by the Council of Deans Advisory Board, May 7, 2018

*If any date falls on a weekend/holiday the recommendation(s) will apply to the following business day.

The AAMC Application and Acceptance Protocols for Admissions Officers

The AAMC application policies are established protocols for applicants and admissions officers.

The AAMC recommends the following guidelines to ensure that MD and MD-PhD applicants are afforded timely notification of the outcome of their applications and timely access to available first-year positions and that schools and programs are able to reasonably anticipate accepted applicant matriculation in order to avoid unfilled positions in their entering classes. For the purposes of these protocols, *matriculation* means that a student has begun a pre-matriculation program, attended orientation immediately preceding enrollment, or enrolled in classes at a medical school.

These protocols are often referred to as "Traffic Rules" by admissions officers and prehealth advisors. These recommendations are distributed for the information of prospective MD and MD-PhD students, their advisors, and personnel at the medical schools and programs to which they have applied, and they are offered in the spirit of undertaking the admission process with the high degree of integrity expected of the medical profession. These guidelines are not intended to supersede the policies, timelines, or discretion of the individual schools or programs. The AAMC understands that an individual's circumstances (e.g., delays in receiving financial aid offer or other compelling personal reasons) may warrant exception from one or more of the following protocols, and defers to each school's judgment in such cases.

The AAMC recommends that each MD or MD-PhD granting school or program:

1. Comply with established procedures to:
   a. Annually publish, amend, and adhere to its application, acceptance, and admission procedures.
   b. Abide by all conditions of participation agreements with application services (if using).

2. Promptly communicate admissions decisions:
   a. By October 1, notify Early Decision applicants and the American Medical College Application Service® (AMCAS®) of Early Decision Program (EDP) admission actions.
   b. From October 15 to March 15, notify AMCAS within five business days of all admission actions, either written or verbal, that have been communicated to an applicant.
   c. From March 16 to April 30, notify AMCAS within two business days of all admissions acceptance, withdrawal, or deferral actions, either written or verbal, that have been communicated to an applicant. All admission actions are listed and defined on the AAMC website.
   d. From May 1 to the first day of class, notify AMCAS of all admission actions within 24 hours.
   e. Notify AMCAS of each student's matriculation within 24 hours.
   f. An acceptance action is defined as the point at which a medical school communicates a written or verbal acceptance offer to an applicant.
   g. An acceptance offer to any dual-degree program that occurs after an initial acceptance should follow the above timelines.

3. Notify all Regular MD program applicants of their acceptance on or after October 15* of each admission cycle, but no earlier. Schools and programs may notify applicants of admission decisions other than acceptance prior to October 15.

4. By March 15 of the matriculation year, issue a number of acceptance offers at least equal to the expected number of students in its first-year entering class and report those acceptance actions to AMCAS.

5. On or before April 30, permit **ALL** applicants (except for EDP applicants):
   a. A minimum of two weeks to respond to their acceptance offer.
   b. To hold acceptance offers or a waitlist position from any other schools or programs without penalty (i.e., scholarships).

6. After April 30:
   a. Permit all applicants:
      1. A minimum of five business days to respond to an acceptance offer. This may be reduced to a minimum of two business days within 30 days of the start of orientation.
      2. To submit a statement of intent, a deposit, or both.
   b. Recognize and respect the challenges of applicants with multiple acceptance offers, applicants who have not yet received an acceptance offer, and applicants who have not yet been informed about financial aid opportunities at schools to which they have been accepted.

7. In addition to any condition included in a school's offer letter, after April 30, each school may exercise its school-specific procedures to confirm an accepted applicant's intention to matriculate or to ensure that it fills each seat in its entering class. If a school is unable to confirm an applicant's intention to matriculate, the school may choose to rescind the acceptance.

8. Each school's initial deposit(s) should not exceed $100 and (except for EDP applicants) and should be refundable at least until April 30. If the applicant enrolls at the school, the school should credit the deposit toward tuition.

9. Making an offer of admission to an applicant who has already matriculated at another school could result in the other school having an unfilled slot in its class. Each school is encouraged to take reasonable measures, including asking applicants under consideration whether they have already matriculated at another medical school, and carefully consider that information when deciding whether to make an offer to an applicant.

10. Each school, consistent with its own privacy policies, should appropriately safeguard information related to an individual's application for admission or financial aid.

11. Each school should treat all letters of evaluation submitted in support of an application as **confidential**, except in those states with applicable laws to the contrary. The contents of a letter of evaluation should not be revealed to an applicant at any time.

Approved by the Council of Deans Advisory Board, May 7, 2018

*If any date falls on a weekend/holiday the recommendation(s) will apply to the following business day.

AMCAS Reports Provided to Medical Schools

To help medical schools adhere to the application and acceptance protocols, AMCAS provides the following reports to schools.

School Acceptance Report. Schools begin receiving this report on September 1, and it includes a list of all accepted applicants at that school. On February 10, this report also begins to include "multiple acceptance data." This means that if a medical school accepts you, they will be able to see a list of any other schools that have also accepted you. Schools can never see how many schools you applied to or if you received a rejection from other schools.

National Acceptance Report. This report is released beginning on April 1 and includes a list of all AMCAS applicants who have been granted at least one acceptance. If an applicant has more than one acceptance, all schools are listed. After October 31, this report also includes the applicant's school of matriculation.

Joint Acceptance Report. This report is also available beginning on April 1. It only includes applicants who are accepted by more than one school. A school viewing this report will see a list of their accepted applicants who are also holding acceptances at one or more other schools. This report also includes applicants with admission actions of deferral, withdrawn after acceptance, and rescinded acceptance.

It's important to keep in mind that:

- Schools can never see how many schools you applied to

- If you're accepted, schools can see other schools that also accepted you starting on February 10 of the application year

- After April 30 of the application year, schools can follow their own policies on how to handle applicants who continue to hold more than one acceptance

Worksheets at the end of chapters in this guide are available in fillable PDF format at *aamc.org/msar-resources*.

Be sure that you're familiar with your school's policy on letters of evaluation. It may provide a committee or composite letter on your behalf. If you're responsible for selecting individuals to write your letters of evaluation, you should look for someone who knows you well and can speak to your readiness for medical school. These letters can be very valuable, so you should be thoughtful in selecting who you ask to write on your behalf.

How to choose an appropriate letter writer and keep track of your interactions with them

Maintain a journal or log that indicates where you've worked and volunteered and what classes you've taken. It's important to keep track of the faculty members and supervisors you work with because those people will likely be able to write you a strong letter of evaluation when it comes time to apply. Keep notes about time spent working on particular projects so you can remember what you did. When you finish working with a particular person, you can go ahead and ask them to write you a reference letter.

Letter writer's name	Why this person would be a good advocate for me	Contact info	Letter complete?
Dr. Nelson	Can speak to my research and writing experience from biology lab	email@school.edu	❏ Yes!
_____	_____ _____ _____	_____ _____ _____	❏ Yes!
_____	_____ _____ _____	_____ _____ _____	❏ Yes!
_____	_____ _____ _____	_____ _____ _____	❏ Yes!

CHAPTER 8

The Admission Decision

What most admissions committees want you to understand is that we consider many elements simultaneously and that we are searching for candidates who fit our institutional missions. Take time to consider your personal mission and how it aligns with each school before you apply. Identify aspects of your education that are important to you, and focus on schools that share your values and what you seek.

Beyond the usual preparatory elements of course work, MCAT scores, health care exposure, leadership, service, and research are the unique perspectives that students bring. Growth and grit are essential to strong applications and your success in medical school. Candidates who demonstrate growth outside their comfort zones are usually able to write and reflect in more meaningful ways because they have challenged themselves. Committees appreciate your showing us those qualities through your preparation, but we need you to do more than simply tell us what you accomplished. Share how your experiences shaped you, about the new ideas and people you encountered in your premed journey, and how you truly vetted your decision to pursue a career entirely dedicated to meeting the needs of others. The best way to tell us about your passions, motivations, and commitments is to demonstrate them through your actions.

To showcase your strengths and passions, you must authentically know yourself. Spend a significant amount of time reflecting on and interrogating your motivations. Be able to explain with personal passion and conviction why you want to be a physician. This defined purpose will carry you through medical school. If you find yourself repeating motivations that generally apply to everyone ("I like people, and I like science"), I urge you to return to the introspection process. If you

Sunny Nakae, MSW, PhD
Assistant Dean for Admissions,
Recruitment, and Student Life
Assistant Professor of Medical Education
Loyola University Chicago
Stritch School of Medicine

are unable to craft a personally meaningful motivation, consider seeking additional experiences that will challenge you.

Professional training is not a race. Admissions committees recognize and value the tremendous diversity of identities and journeys among candidates. Schools may have different missions, but all value diversity among their learners and in the future physician workforce. Committees are drawn to leaders and change agents. We get excited assessing applications that evidence tremendous growth, leadership, and advocacy for others. Medicine is a tough road, and we pursue candidates with the deep conviction that there's nowhere else they would rather be.

Holistic Review of Medical School Applicants

What does holistic review mean, and how does it affect the admission review process?

Holistic review is a flexible, individualized way of assessing an applicant. The review considers a balance of an applicant's experiences, attributes, and academic metrics (E-A-M) and, when taken together, how the individual may contribute value as a medical student and future physician. When admissions committees select individual applicants, they intentionally try to create a broadly diverse class to help fulfill their school's mission.

Each medical school's admissions office evaluates applicants based on the mission, goals, and diversity interests of that institution. Admissions committees must decide which applicants will best serve the needs of their patients, the community, and the medical profession at large. They seek a broadly diverse student body because diversity of backgrounds and perspectives has consistently been shown to drive educational and professional excellence. Schools look for applicants who have developed a track record that demonstrates the knowledge, skills, attitudes, and behaviors that will best prepare them to navigate challenges and thrive as both learners and physicians. Depending on its mission, one school might look for applicants who demonstrate service to communities underserved by the current health care system, while another may seek applicants who have shown creativity and independent productivity in scholarly activities.

Admissions officers carefully review a multitude of criteria—rather than focusing on just one or two facets— to gain an appreciation of the "whole" person. Many applicants believe that admissions officers weigh high GPAs and MCAT® scores above all else. While these academic metrics are important components of the admission decision, they are only one part of the overall package. An applicant's ability to balance multiple priorities and responsibilities as well as the resilience they've shown in handling various issues are considered along with grades and MCAT scores. This helps explain why there are many cases in which a high-scoring student with a near-perfect GPA may not get into medical school, and why others with scores and grades below the average do.

Admission decisions involve more than academic metrics.

Experiences

Your experiences convey a lot about your interests, responsibilities, capabilities, and knowledge. As a result, medical schools take a close look at what you've learned from where you've been up to this stage in your life. It helps them gauge not only how likely you are to be successful in their programs, but also to what degree you'll support their mission and contribute as a physician.

Chapter 2, on undergraduate preparation, mentioned how important your extracurricular activities may be to an admissions committee—and not just those clubs and organizations within your college, but also outside of school. Your experiences—particularly those related to medicine or research—are an important component that affects your competitiveness as a candidate. For instance, if you are balancing a 20-to-30-hour-a-week job to pay for school while attending classes or have responsibilities caring for a younger sibling or elderly relative, those experiences are important to share with admissions committees. They communicate information about your different attributes and provide additional context for interpreting your grades. Your experiences—and the insights you gained from them—also help admissions committees identify what's unique about you and how you may contribute to their school and the practice of medicine.

Beyond that, the degree to which you contributed to and participated in these activities is vital. Medical schools value a demonstration of true commitment, so if you've made a significant contribution to or impact on an organization or taken on increasing levels of responsibility, you'll want to make that clear to the admissions committee. They're interested not only in what you've done, but how you think those experiences have influenced who you are and what you want to do. A series of short-term involvements (volunteering a day here, spending an afternoon there, and so forth) does not really convey a deep interest in the area, and this lack of motivation is transparent to admissions officials. They're looking for substantial, committed participation in areas that are truly important to you. Only then are they able to gain some insights into your real interests and judge how well your goals and their missions align.

Again, the mission of each school will play a large part in how your experience is evaluated. For example, institutions whose goal is to increase the number of physicians practicing in underserved areas will focus attention on the summer you spent volunteering in a free clinic or doing rural or urban community outreach on health promotion. In general, medical schools especially value community and volunteer experience related to the health care field.

Concept of "Distance Traveled"

Here's another thing to consider: Admissions officers are likely to place significance on any obstacles or hardships you've overcome to get to this point in your education. This concept, known as "distance traveled," refers to those life challenges you've faced and conquered. Medical schools view these instances as admirable experiences indicative of some very positive traits, such as resilience and persistence. As with other experiences, you can help the admissions committee better understand and appreciate your unique contributions by not only describing the experiences, but also describing how they have helped influence you and your desire to be a physician.

Experiences likely to be important to admissions committees:

- Serving as the primary caregiver for an ill family member
- Overcoming obstacles or hardships

- Being employed (especially if medically related)
- Participating in research

- Working, volunteering, or shadowing in a health care setting
- Participating in and leading community-based or volunteer organizations

Attributes

Admissions committees want to know if you have what it takes to become a competent and compassionate doctor. This includes the ability to master the science and medicine behind it all, of course, but it also requires that you have some key personal attributes. They use various methods to determine whether you have those attributes. While personal experiences such as volunteering for three consecutive summers at a medical clinic certainly convey dedication and help demonstrate your proficiency in these areas, admissions committees will look to your personal statement, letters of evaluation, and interviews to gauge whether you have the desire to build on these experiences in medical school.

Are you empathetic? Do you have integrity? Can you communicate effectively and with people different from yourself? Traits such as these are necessary to develop into the kind of physician needed for the future.

Examples of attributes likely to be important to admissions committees:

- Adaptability
- Critical thinking
- Integrity
- Logical reasoning
- Oral communication skills
- Resilience

- Personal maturity
- Reliability
- Self-discipline
- Work habits
- Compassion

- Cultural competence
- Intellectual curiosity
- Motivation for medicine
- Persistence
- Professionalism

Medical schools analyze a broad range of attributes, including those related to the applicant's skills and abilities, personal and professional characteristics, and demographic factors.

- **Skills and abilities** could include active listening, critical thinking, and multilingual ability.

- **Personal and professional characteristics** could include resilience, intellectual curiosity, and empathy.

- **Demographic factors** could include socioeconomic status, race, and gender.

In addition to these general qualities, medical schools give weight to specific characteristics that align with their missions. Examples could include research inquisitiveness, empathy, teamwork, curiosity, and a desire for knowledge about health care delivery systems.

Academic Metrics

Admissions committees need to determine whether you have the academic skills and knowledge necessary to succeed in medical school. Committee members will consider your academic record and MCAT scores to measure your knowledge and abilities objectively.

Academic History

Your academic history helps admissions committees determine whether your study skills, persistence, course of study, and grades predict success at their medical school. Committee members carefully review your college transcript and consider:

- Grades earned in each course and lab

- Grade trends in the last two years of schooling

- Number of credit hours carried in each academic period

- Distribution of coursework among the biological, physical, and social sciences and the humanities

- Need for remediation of unsatisfactory academic work

- Number of incomplete grades and course withdrawals

- Number of years taken to complete the degree program

- The amount of advanced coursework completed in addition to the standard prerequisites and requirements

MCAT Scores

Admissions committees can better predict success when they add MCAT scores into the mix. That's because there can be significant differences in grading scales and standards from college to college, and MCAT scores provide a standardized measure by which to compare applicants. In fact, the ability of admissions officers to predict who will be successful in the first two years of their programs increases by as much as 50% (gauging by first- and second-year medical school grades) when they look at MCAT scores in conjunction with undergraduate GPAs rather than grades alone.

As a result, the better your grades and the higher your scores, the more likely you are to be accepted. It is important to remember that there's still a wide range of MCAT scores and GPAs found among accepted applicants and that those are used in conjunction with other factors, as discussed earlier in this chapter.

Making the Evaluation

Admissions committees gauge all three of these areas—experiences, attributes, and academic metrics—and how they relate to each other in several ways. Although each medical school establishes its own criteria, schools usually prefer applicants who balanced science and humanities coursework, carried respectable course loads, and, generally speaking, earned 3.0–4.0 GPAs (on a 4.0 scale).

Several elements within the application process speak to your experiences and attributes. Your personal statement, as mentioned in Chapter 7, gives you the opportunity to tell committee members about your extracurricular activities, distance traveled, volunteer efforts, and medical-related work experience. The personal attributes that accompany these activities can often be inferred. For example, a role as an officer in a school club conveys leadership experience. Working in a medical clinic summer after summer demonstrates motivation for medicine. A long history of volunteering with fundraisers for cancer research suggests teamwork and compassion. Applicants can speak to these experiences in their statements and during interviews to further underscore these connections.

Your letters of evaluation, also described in Chapter 7, attest to your personal attributes. Ask your professors and advisor (and other evaluators) to address your persistence, strong work habits, and self-discipline. (The faculty and administrative staff at your undergraduate school will know how to craft a letter, but for others, you might want to suggest a few key concepts.)

Then there are the academic metrics. As you may know, your academic record is part of your AMCAS application and includes both your college transcript(s) and MCAT scores. From there, committee members can determine whether you have the grades, range of coursework, and foundation of knowledge they seek in their successful applicants.

Schools consider your experiences, attributes, and academic metrics in combination. Together, they give shape to what you, as an applicant, may contribute to their medical school and to health care at large. So keep this in mind: It's not only about what you did and what you know, but it's also about who you are and what you bring to the learning environment and the medical profession.

The Interview Is Key

If you've been invited to an interview, you should feel confident because you've already impressed your reviewers with your strong personal statement, background, letters of evaluation, and academic history. The interview day gives you a chance to tour the medical school's facility and meet the students, faculty, and staff you may be interacting with for the next several years. Take this opportunity to assess the culture and learning environment and explore whether the school might be a good fit for you. Now, you have an opportunity to "shine." Medical schools usually interview significantly more applicants than their class size, and this is why the interview is likely to be the number one determining factor at this point in the admission process. Other factors include how you interact with others and how you react to stressful questions.

The fact that interviews are given at all is a significant distinction of medical schools because some professional schools don't require them. The medical school interview attests to the degree to which admissions officers seek—and medical schools value—qualities and characteristics such as empathy, self-awareness, communication ability, and interpersonal skills that can best be judged in a direct interview situation. You can take these steps to ensure you're prepared for it.

Know the Basics

Whether it's for a new job or for a seat in a medical school's entering class, certain similarities exist in all interviewing situations. A good start is to review any interviewing books in your school's library or prehealth advisor's office, find out whether your advisor or premed club offers a mock-interview session, and search online for tips and interview resources. The Aspiring Docs® library offers two fact sheets that describe the most common types of interviews and tips on how to prepare yourself. Check out the fact sheets at *aamc.org/aspiringdocs*.

Know What Type of Interview to Expect

It helps to be ready for several different interview formats. At some schools, interviews are held with individual admissions committee members; at others, group interviews are the norm. While most interviews are held on the medical school campus, some schools have designated interviewers in different geographic regions to minimize time and expense for applicants. (Information about a school's interview policies and procedures is usually provided to applicants in the initial stages of the selection process.) Check the Medical School Admission Requirements™ website to find the type of interviews offered, such as one-on-one, panel, multiple mini interview, and video interview (*aamc.org/msar*).

Be Comfortable With Different Interviewing Styles

You probably have had some experience interviewing for summer and part-time jobs (and possibly for your undergraduate school), so it won't surprise you that interviewers have their own styles and follow different formats. Some interviewers follow a structured design, asking questions from a predetermined list and assigning numeric scores to each answer. Others prefer a more free-flowing arrangement and provide the applicant with a greater degree of open input. Increasingly, schools are using the multiple mini interview (MMI), which typically consists of 6 to 10 very short interviews that revolve around a specific scenario. The MMI assesses communication skills, specifically verbal and nonverbal skills that cannot be measured using standardized written exams or reviewing coursework transcripts.

For more information, review the MMI fact sheet at *students-residents.aamc.org/applying-medical-school/article/what-its-participate-multiple-mini-interviews-mmis*.

Do Your Research

Being able to speak knowledgeably about the medical school shows that you're interested and invested in this particular program. Investigate the school thoroughly by reviewing its profile on the Medical School Admission Requirements website (*aamc.org/msar*), the school's website, the information packet sent to you, and any articles you can find. Your time is limited, so don't waste it by asking questions already answered on their website, in their materials, or on the Medical School Admission Requirements website. Try to talk with current students to get an accurate sense of what the school is like from a student perspective. You'll want to impress your interviewer not only with your potential for success, but also with your interest in the specific institution. You can demonstrate these qualities through your answers to the interviewer's questions, as well as by the questions you ask.

Be Ready to Ask Questions

There will come a point in your interview when you'll be asked if you have any questions, and it's an opportunity you don't want to pass up. Not only can you clarify any remaining issues, but you'll have another way to demonstrate your commitment, astuteness, and interest in that particular school. With that in mind, you'll want to prepare two or three questions specific to that school. Need a way to generate ideas? Check out the AAMC's "Thirty-Five Questions I Wish I Had Asked" at *aamc.org/35questions*.

Practice

Most admissions committee members are experienced interviewers who want to learn about the "real" person you are. Be honest and open during your meeting and do not try to just give the answers you think the interviewer wants to hear. Try to keep the interview conversational. If you're apprehensive about the process, asking a trusted advisor or friend to conduct mock interviews with you can help build your confidence.

Remember, the interview is an opportunity to discuss your personal history and motivation for pursuing a career in medicine. It also gives you a chance to address any aspects of your application that merit emphasis or explanation. Be sure to present yourself in the best possible light by preparing thoroughly for your meeting. Think about how you conduct yourself among current students and staff during informal meetings, too. Every interaction can create an impression of who you are, and how you present yourself usually comes up during a post-interview discussion.

A Few Last Reminders for Your Interview Day

When it comes to what to wear, a good rule of thumb is to dress for the job you seek. In short, look professional. Your interview is likely to be coupled with a tour of the campus, so be sure to wear shoes and an outfit that you're comfortable walking in.

Your interview day is a long one. You'll be doing a lot of talking and meeting numerous people. It's okay to bring a water bottle or drink with you. It's very important to be aware that everyone on campus you encounter is someone who can give feedback about you—positive and negative. Be sure to use good manners, be courteous to all, and show your enthusiasm. Lastly, keep your phone out of sight and on silent. You should not have it out at any time during the interview or campus tour. Remember, the people you speak with are not only evaluating your academic potential, but they're also seeing how you conduct yourself professionally and whether you're a good fit for their medical school.

Your Interview Rights and Responsibilities

Although interviewers are instructed by admissions officers and guided by federal statutes on what are unfair or discriminatory preadmission inquiries, there may be an occasion when an interviewer asks an inappropriate question. (See examples in box at right.)

You have the right not to answer what you sense is an inappropriate question. If such a question is asked, try to relax and provide a thoughtful and articulate response (two essential characteristics of a good physician). You may also respectfully decline to answer the question and explain that you were advised not to answer questions that you sensed were inappropriate.

You have the responsibility to report being asked an inappropriate question to help prevent further occurrences. Medical schools have the responsibility to establish procedures that enable applicants to report such incidents in a confidential manner.

Medical schools should inform you of these procedures prior to interviews and assure you that reporting an incident will not bias your evaluation.

If a medical school did not inform you of its procedures and an incident occurs, use these guidelines. If possible, report in confidence to an admissions officer during the interview day the interviewer's name and the interview question(s) asked. Otherwise, email this information to an admissions officer within 24 hours of the interview, noting the date and time of the incident. Furthermore, you have the right to ask if another interview is deemed necessary to ensure an unbiased evaluation of your application to that medical school.

Some interviewers use the interview to assess how well you function under stress and may purposely ask challenging questions to observe how you respond under pressure. How you communicate will be a critical part of the encounter; however, this does not give an interviewer the right to ask you inappropriate questions in their attempt to challenge you during the interview.

Examples of inappropriate questions:

Q. *What is your race, ethnicity, religion, sexual orientation, political affiliation, marital status, opinion on abortion and/or euthanasia, income, value of your home, credit score, etc.?*

Q. *Are you planning on having children during medical school?*

Q. *Do you have any disabilities?*

Q. *Will you require special accommodations?*

Q. *Have you ever been arrested?*

Q. *Have you ever done drugs?*

Q. *How old are you?*

Sample responses to inappropriate questions:

Q. *What are your plans for expanding your family during medical school?*

A. Can you please clarify your question? I want to make sure that I'm providing information that is most relevant to my candidacy.

Q. *Have you ever done drugs?*

A. I am uncomfortable discussing my medical history and possible use of prescription medication.

Worksheets at the end of chapters in this guide are available in fillable PDF format at *aamc.org/msar-resources*.

Core Competencies and Anatomy of an Applicant

While each medical school has its own process for reviewing candidates, many medical schools use the **15 Core Competencies for Entering Medical Students**, which has been endorsed by the AAMC Group on Student Affairs (GSA) Committee on Admissions (COA). These competencies provide a framework to consider when communicating how your work, activities, and life experiences demonstrate your readiness for medical school. Successful medical school applicants are able to show that they possess skills, knowledge, and capabilities in the 15 defined areas shown in Table 8.1.

Table 8.1. Core Competencies for Entering Medical Students Endorsed by the AAMC Group on Student Affairs Committee on Admissions

Preprofessional Competencies	Thinking and Reasoning Competencies	Science Competencies
• Service Orientation • Social Skills • Cultural Competence • Teamwork • Oral Communication • Ethical Responsibility to Self and Others • Reliability and Dependability • Resilience and Adaptability • Capacity for Improvement	• Critical Thinking • Quantitative Reasoning • Scientific Inquiry • Written Communication	• Living Systems • Human Behavior

To help explain the competencies and provide real examples, the AAMC created Anatomy of an Applicant (*students-residents.aamc.org/applying-medical-school/preparing-med-school/anatomy-applicant/*), a resource that shares the pathways of medical students, along with commentary from their prehealth advisors and the admissions officers who accepted them. This resource was developed in direct response to inquiries from applicants, prehealth advisors, and admissions officers who asked the AAMC for help in better understanding how applicants can convey their aptitude in the core competencies. It provides guidance on how the core competencies could be developed and demonstrated through an applicant's experiences in preparation for medical school.

The work and activities you are already involved with, and your life experiences, likely demonstrate these competencies. For example, you can show competency in scientific inquiry by excelling in scientific research, or you can illustrate competency in service orientation by leading a service trip. And as you'll see in the Anatomy of an Applicant student profiles (*students-residents.aamc.org/applying-medical-school/preparing-med-school/anatomy-applicant/demonstrate-the-core-competencies/*), one experience can offer evidence of proficiency across multiple competencies. These profiles share the personal stories of medical students—their path to medical school and what they identify as their strongest competencies. Anatomy of an Applicant also includes competency definitions, parts of an application and what they tell schools about you, and self-assessment worksheets.

As you research the medical schools you're interested in attending, use this worksheet to keep track of questions you think you may want to ask during your interview. Print or save this page for individual schools, and review it the night before your interview or bring it with you. You can find many questions here: *aamc.org/35questions*.

Name of Medical School: _____

Type of Interview: _____

Date of Interview: _____

Questions about:

1. Curriculum _____

   _____

   _____

2. Student Involvement _____

   _____

   _____

3. Special Programs _____

   _____

   _____

4. Financial Aid _____

   _____

   _____

5. Facilities _____

   _____

   _____

6. Academic Evaluations _____

   _____

   _____

7. Student Support _____

   _____

   _____

8. Residency Placements _____

   _____

   _____

9. Other _____

   _____

CHAPTER 9

Applicant and Acceptee Data

> Leave it to medical school applications to incite an identity crisis unlike I'd ever experienced before! As applicants, we're forced to reflect on the level of honesty we portray to ourselves, and there's no hiding from our unmet expectations or insecurities. Your personal statement, scores, and transcript are all on full display and at the mercy of an admissions committee, ready for careful dissection.
>
> There was little reason for me to be optimistic. By all traditional objective measures of evaluation, I wasn't a competitive applicant, and I wasn't exactly doing myself any favors, either: I was a reapplicant. I sat for and survived the MCAT exam five times, and my GPA could be found on the lower end of the distribution curve. Solely based on numbers, I had wrongly written myself off, jumping to conclusions about how I would be labeled and perceived, without considering anything else I had to offer. Yet, with each interview invite, I was proven incorrect. My ultimate acceptance served as a reminder that the admissions process is not as one-dimensional as I once thought—it credits those who have overcome barriers, demonstrated resilience, and been successful despite circumstances.
>
> Navigating the application process is a unique and personal experience for everyone. We come into it with a preconceived notion of what an ideal applicant is and isn't, subscribing to a checklist of standards that's not necessarily universal or realistic for all. Numbers inform but do not define. Remember what makes you, you. That'll take you farther than any score ever will.

Luis E. Seija
MD Candidate
Texas A&M University
College of Medicine
Class of 2019

This chapter summarizes data about the entire applicant pool, as well as about accepted applicants and people who weren't accepted for the 2017 entering class. The data, from the AAMC Applicant Matriculant File, are accurate as of October 19, 2017. In the figures:

- "All applicants" refers to all applicants to the 2017 entering class
- "Accepted applicants" refers to those accepted to at least one medical school
- "Not-accepted applicants" refers to those not accepted to any medical school

We include data related to performance on the MCAT® exam, undergraduate grade point average (GPA) and major, sex, age, medical/clinical and other experiences, and race and ethnicity.

A Quick Look at the 2017 Entering Class

- In 2016–2017, 51,680 people applied to the 2017 entering class at all MD-granting medical schools in the United States.

- With the introduction of the new exam in 2015, there was some concern that some groups of examinees would be more reluctant than others to take the exam, but examinees from various backgrounds took the exam in the same proportions as in previous years.

- By the fall of 2017, 22,266 applicants had been offered an acceptance to at least one medical school, and 21,339 accepted applicants had matriculated. A small number of accepted applicants—927—chose not to matriculate in 2017.

The accepted applicants had broad ranges of MCAT scores and undergraduate GPAs and a wide variety of personal characteristics and life experiences. Both male and female applicants were distributed across numerous racial and ethnic groups. Although a few applied through the Early Decision Program, the vast majority used the regular application process.

Performance on the MCAT Exam

Figure 9.1 summarizes the overall performance of the 2017 applicants who submitted scores from the new MCAT exam. The figure shows that these 2017 applicants achieved total scores from 472 to 528; the median score for applicants for 2017 was 505. Accepted applicants had total scores ranging from 482 to 528; about 16 accepted applicants had total scores of 487 or below (an average of almost 121 on each section of the test). The total MCAT score most commonly achieved by accepted applicants was 511.

It's possible that some prospective applicants saw the launch of the new MCAT exam as an opportunity. As applicants and admissions committees were establishing new conventions for weighing those new MCAT scores in relation to other applicant data, students with a wide range of MCAT scores and undergraduate GPAs applied for admission to medical school in 2017.

No score on a single MCAT section and no total MCAT score will "guarantee" admission to medical school. Figure 9.1 shows that a substantial number of applicants with total MCAT scores of 512 and above were not accepted. This finding reveals the importance of factors other than MCAT performance—including undergraduate academic performance and a variety of personal characteristics and experiences—in the medical student selection process.

Undergraduate Grade Point Average

Figure 9.2 presents information about the undergraduate academic performance of 2017 applicants. All applicants had cumulative total undergraduate GPAs from just under 2.0 to 4.0, and most were between 3.75 and 4.0. Accepted applicants' total undergraduate GPAs ranged from just over 2.0 to 4.0, and 86 had total undergraduate GPAs of 2.75 or below. The turning point where more applicants were accepted than rejected began with a GPA between 3.75 and 4.0.

As is the case with the MCAT data, the GPA data in Figure 9.2 show that no undergraduate GPA ensures admission to medical school. Although applicants with total GPAs in the range of 3.75 to 4.0 were more likely to be accepted to medical school, a significant number of such applicants were not accepted. Again, these findings underscore the importance of other factors, such as personal characteristics and life experiences, in the medical student selection process.

Figure 9.1. MCAT total score distribution, 2017 applicants.

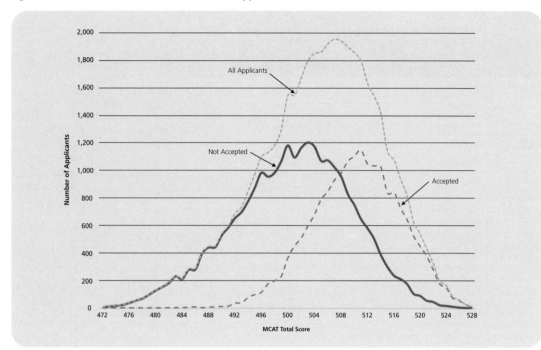

Source: AAMC Data Warehouse as of October 19, 2017.

Figure 9.2. Grade point average (GPA) total distribution, 2017 applicants.

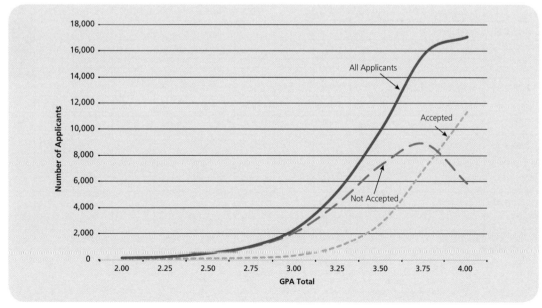

Source: AAMC Data Warehouse as of October 19, 2017.

Table 9.1. MCAT Total Scores and Total GPAs of Applicants and Acceptees, 2016–2017 (Aggregated)

GPA Total	Acceptees (Accs), Applicants (Apps), and Percentage of Applicants Accepted	MCAT Total									
		472–485	486–489	490–493	494–497	498–501	502–505	506–509	510–513	514–517	518–528
3.80–4.00	Acceptees	2	7	54	203	627	1,491	2,368	2,718	2,477	2,378
	Applicants	97	198	483	982	1,850	2,802	3,585	3,580	2,934	2,679
	Accs/Apps	2.1%	3.5%	11.2%	20.7%	33.9%	53.2%	66.1%	75.9%	84.4%	88.8%
3.60–3.79	Acceptees	1	7	57	230	613	1,193	1,799	1,949	1,382	847
	Applicants	255	454	892	1,596	2,487	3,220	3,459	2,924	1,821	1,026
	Accs/Apps	0.4%	1.5%	6.4%	14.4%	24.6%	37.0%	52.0%	66.7%	75.9%	82.6%
3.40–3.59	Acceptees	5	5	47	177	458	749	947	968	579	317
	Applicants	406	590	1,100	1,733	2,308	2,626	2,454	1,808	936	456
	Accs/Apps	1.2%	0.8%	4.3%	10.2%	19.8%	28.5%	38.6%	53.5%	61.9%	69.5%
3.20–3.39	Acceptees	3	5	29	111	247	373	404	357	249	90
	Applicants	483	592	995	1,356	1,575	1,653	1,317	911	452	166
	Accs/Apps	0.6%	0.8%	2.9%	8.2%	15.7%	22.6%	30.7%	39.2%	55.1%	54.2%
3.00–3.19	Acceptees	3	5	8	50	123	174	149	137	67	31
	Applicants	511	516	692	850	883	836	628	416	157	76
	Accs/Apps	0.6%	1.0%	1.2%	5.9%	13.9%	20.8%	23.7%	32.9%	42.7%	40.8%
2.80–2.99	Acceptees	4	3	8	18	35	60	49	34	18	7
	Applicants	448	350	418	440	436	339	243	125	71	17
	Accs/Apps	0.9%	0.9%	1.9%	4.1%	8.0%	17.7%	20.2%	27.2%	25.4%	41.2%
2.60–2.79	Acceptees	1	1	1	8	14	22	17	9	9	8
	Applicants	309	223	249	248	203	136	99	59	25	14
	Accs/Apps	0.3%	0.4%	0.4%	3.2%	6.9%	16.2%	17.2%	15.3%	36.0%	57.1%
2.40–2.59	Acceptees	0	2	1	5	4	8	9	4	3	0
	Applicants	218	108	108	109	77	46	43	25	7	2
	Accs/Apps	0.0%	1.9%	0.9%	4.6%	5.2%	17.4%	20.9%	16.0%	42.9%	0.0%
2.20–2.39	Acceptees	0	0	0	0	2	5	1	2	0	1
	Applicants	134	47	42	41	27	24	20	11	0	
	Accs/Apps	0.0%	0.0%	0.0%	0.0%	7.4%	20.8%	5.0%	18.2%		33.3%
2.00–2.19	Acceptees	0	0	0	0	0	0	0	0	0	1
	Applicants	73	25	20	16	8	8	3	3	0	1
	Accs/Apps	0.0%	0.0%	0.0%	0.0%	0.0%	0.0%	0.0%	0.0%		100.0%
1.41–1.99	Acceptees	0	0	1	0	0	0	0	0	0	0
	Applicants	35	12	9	6	1	2	1	1	0	0
	Accs/Apps	0.0%	0.0%	11.1%	0.0%	0.0%	0.0%	0.0%	0.0%	—	—

Note: Percentage accepted = ☐ <25% ☐ 25%–49% ■ 50%–74% ■ 75%–100%

Source: AAMC Data Warehouse: Applicant Matriculant File as of October 19, 2017.

MCAT Score

Table 9.1 combines MCAT scores and undergraduate GPA for all 2017 applicants to medical school who submitted scores from the new exam. Note that these results are presented without regard to any of the other selection factors. If the data don't reflect your particular circumstances, please go to *aamc.org/data/ facts* to see acceptance rates for specific demographic groups.

Sex

Figure 9.3 presents information about the number and sex of the entire applicant pool and accepted applicants for the 1992 to 2017 entering classes. In 2017, the applicant pool decreased 2.6% from 2016. Therefore, the largest annual applicant pool during the past 25 years remains the 2016 entering class, a pool of 53,042.

The number of male applicants to the 2017 entering class decreased by 1,192 from the number of male applicants to the previous year's entering class. The number of female applicants to the 2017 class decreased by 179 over the number to the previous year's entering class.

Although the number of accepted applicants remained fairly constant from 1992 to 2002, it started to increase in 2003, from 17,542 in that year to a high of 22,266 in 2017. The number of accepted male applicants has fluctuated since 1992, with a low of 8,810 in 2003 and a high of 11,271 in 2015. The number of accepted female applicants has increased, with small fluctuations, from a low of 7,255 in the 1994 entering class to a high of 11,287 in 2017. The significant gaps between male and female applicants for the 1994 entering class (7,426) and the 1995 entering class (7,034) have lessened; 553 and 301 more females than males applied to the 2003 and 2004 entering classes, respectively. In 2005, 122 more males than females applied. In 2017, 458 more males than females applied to medical school. During the same time span, the gaps between accepted male and accepted female applicants decreased. Accepted male applicants outnumbered accepted female applicants by 2,951 for the 1992 entering class, but for the 2017 entering class, 321 more females than males were accepted.

Figure 9.3. Applicants by sex and acceptance status, 1992–2017.

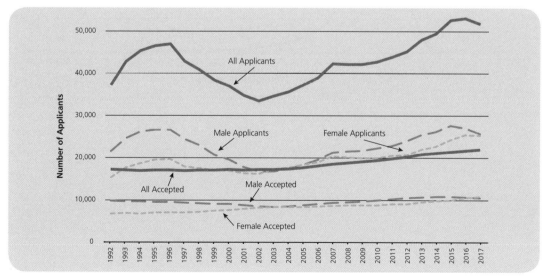

Source: AAMC Data Warehouse as of October 19, 2017.

The national ratio of male to female applicants was 49.2:50.8 for the 2003 entering class, the first time that the number of female applicants to medical school was greater than the number of male applicants. For the 2004 entering class, this trend continued, with a 49.6:50.4 ratio of male to female applicants. For the 2005 entering class, there were once again more male applicants than female applicants, with a male-to-female ratio of 50.2:49.8. This trend continued until 2017, when the number of female applicants outnumbered males (50.4:49.5).

Age

Figure 9.4 shows that the age distribution for all applicants to the 2017 entering class was broad. The applicants between 21 and 28 years of age when they were expected to matriculate totaled 46,993; the number of applicants under 21 was 493; and applicants over 28 numbered 4,194. Figure 9.4 shows a similar finding for accepted applicants to the 2017 entering class; these individuals were between 18 and 53 years of age at the time of expected matriculation.

Figure 9.4. Age distribution, 2017 applicants.

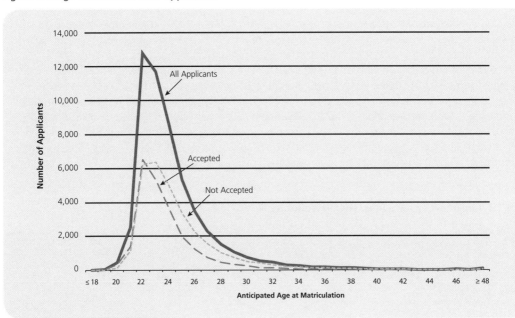

Source: AAMC Data Warehouse as of October 19, 2017.

Applicant and Accepted Applicant Experiences

Figure 9.5 summarizes the volunteer and research experiences of AMCAS® applicants and accepted applicants to the 2017 entering class. The figure clearly shows the increase in the percentage of both applicants and accepted applicants reporting volunteer medical, community service, and research experience since 2002:

- 82% of accepted applicants reported community service and/or volunteer medical or clinical experience, an increase of about 6% since 2002

- 77% of applicants reported community service and/or volunteer medical or clinical experience, an increase of about 4% since 2002

- 85% of accepted applicants reported research and/or lab experience, an increase of about 16% since 2002

- 77% of applicants reported research and/or lab experience, an increase of about 14% since 2002

- 77% of accepted applicants reported nonmedical or nonclinical community service and/or volunteer experience, an increase of about 11% since 2002

- 72% of applicants reported nonmedical or nonclinical community service and/or volunteer experience, an increase of about 10% since 2002

Figure 9.5. Percentage of AMCAS applicants and accepted applicants reporting selected experiences, 2002–2017.

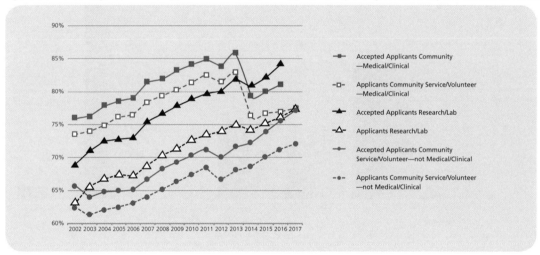

Source: AAMC Data Warehouse as of October 19, 2017.

Self-Identity

Figure 9.6 shows self-reported race and ethnicity data for applicants to the 2014 entering class through the 2017 entering class. Applicants can enter multiple races and ethnicities, so the sum of those shown does not equal the total number of applicants. Also, we couldn't include applicants for whom we have no race and ethnicity data. Additional information for applicants from groups underrepresented in medicine is available in Chapter 4.

Figure 9.6. Distribution of self-identity, all applicants, 2014–2017.*

*Self-identities are reported for U.S. citizens or permanent residents only and may be alone or in combination with some other self-identity.

Source: AAMC Data Warehouse as of October 19, 2017.

CHAPTER 10

You Can Afford Medical School

Attending medical school is an expensive financial investment. Various forms of financial aid are available to help students pay for the cost of a medical education, including scholarships, grants, and federal, institutional, and private loans. A major consideration in my choice of which medical school to attend was the robustness of my financial aid package and an in-depth understanding of living expenses.

Here are my personal recommendations for managing finances in medical school:

- *Get to know your school's financial aid team. It is a critical resource in helping you make the right decisions for your specific financial situation.*

- *Be proactive in getting all your questions related to financial aid answered. If you find yourself confused or overwhelmed, speak with a financial aid counselor—they're there to help guide you.*

- *Track your expenses. In addition to helping you live within your means, tracking expenses is a vital life skill that will serve you well in the future.*

- *Know what you borrowed and who you borrowed from. It sounds basic, but it's essential to know this when it comes time for repayment.*

Ultimately, I relied closely on my school's financial aid office, AAMC online resources, and my personal support system for advice and guidance in financing my medical education. The investment you make in attending medical school is significant, but there are resources and tools and advisors to help you make this daunting process much smoother.

Dipika Gaur
MD Candidate
Rush Medical College
of Rush University
Class of 2021

Building a Strong Financial Plan

You'll need to develop a strategy to cover the costs associated with your education. Don't let the numbers discourage you. There's help available.

When you look at the figures in Table 10.1, the financial challenges may seem overwhelming. Annual tuition, fees, and health insurance for the first year at state medical schools in 2016–2017 averaged about $35,932 for residents and $60,543 for nonresidents; at private schools, the average was $57,492 for residents and $58,895 for nonresidents.

According to recent surveys conducted by the AAMC, 75% of newly graduated MDs have medical school education loans, and 63% reported receiving some degree of help through scholarships, stipends, and

Table 10.1. Tuition, Fees, and Health Insurance for 2017–2018 First-Year Students in U.S. Medical Schools* (in Dollars)

Private Schools			
Student Category	**Range**	**Median**	**Average**
Resident	$24,363–$66,661	$59,605	$57,492
Nonresident	$37,165–$67,480	$60,300	$58,895

Public Schools			
Student Category	**Range**	**Median**	**Average**
Resident	$0**–$53,327	$36,817	$35,932
Nonresident	$0**–$98,538	$62,466	$60,543

*Analysis excludes the Brody School of Medicine at East Carolina University, University of Massachusetts Medical School, Mercer University School of Medicine, University of Mississippi School of Medicine, and Southern Illinois School University of Medicine. These schools do not accept nonresident medical students, and therefore, they do not report nonresident tuition and fees. "Public Schools" excludes Uniformed Services University of Health Sciences, which does not charge tuition or student fees.

**Instead of paying tuition and fees, students at Uniformed Services–Hébert incur a national service obligation.

Source: 2016–2017 AAMC Tuition and Student Fees Questionnaire.

grants (which you don't have to repay). So, it can be done, and it *is* … by tens of thousands of medical students every single year. But first: You'll need a plan.

Before you actually borrow money, it's important that you understand—and adhere to—the basic principles of successful money management. With that in mind, the three basic recommendations that follow should help you build a strong financial foundation.

1. Live Within Your Means

All other efforts to "afford" medical school and handle your monies wisely will be undermined if you don't have a plan of action for your finances. Having a spending plan is the cornerstone of a solid financial foundation. Let's face it, money will be tight during medical school, and a realistic spending plan will be critical to your financial well-being. A well-crafted plan will help you maintain better control of your spending, ensure you cover your essential expenses, and prepare you for unexpected expenses by building an emergency fund.

Creating a budget involves only a few steps:

- Income—document incoming funds, which will likely be in the form of financial aid (loans, scholarships, or grants)

- Expenses—identify outgoing expenses, like rent, food, and tuition

Figure 10.1. Distribution of financial aid among medical students.

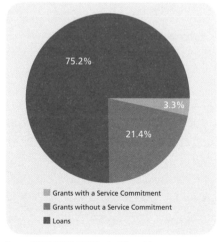

75.2%

3.3%

21.4%

■ Grants with a Service Commitment
■ Grants without a Service Commitment
■ Loans

Source: 2016–2017 LCME Student Financial Aid Questionnaire Part I-B.

- Discretionary income—calculate your discretionary income to see if your spending plan allows you to live within your means

- For assistance in creating a realistic budget, contact the financial aid office of the medical school you're interested in attending. Often, they can provide some approximations of the average amount of student loan monies available to live on and the expected costs of necessities while attending medical school.

Your Total Income — Your Total Expenses = Your Discretionary Income

2. Manage Your Debt Wisely

- Given the costs of medical school, it's understandable that the vast majority of medical students borrow money to fund their education—and, as of 2017, graduate with median education debt of $192,000. The ability to manage debt wisely is important, regardless of one's situation, and it becomes even more critical for you—a prospective medical student—when you consider the degree to which you're likely to rely on loans to help pay for your education.

- Be conscious of the amount you're likely to borrow, and be comfortable knowing that your future income will allow you to repay your student loan debt.

- Educate yourself about various financing possibilities before you arrive at medical school, and diligently search for free money, such as scholarships, grants, and repayment assistance programs.

- Understand your responsibilities—beyond making payments—that come with borrowing student loans. These include knowing what loans you borrowed, where to send payments, and when payments are due. You'll also be responsible for notifying your servicers of any changes to your name, contact information, or enrollment status.

- Stay organized. Maintain accurate financial aid records, copies of application forms, and any related paperwork. This also means opening and reading all mail pertaining to your student loan debt. The MedLoans® Organizer and Calculator is a tool that can help you keep everything organized. Every accepted medical school student is given access to this free tool, found at *aamc.org/medloans*.

- Build a good credit score by meeting your financial obligations. In doing so, you'll strengthen your ability to qualify for and obtain attractive interest rates for credit-based loans, land a job, and rent an apartment. For more information, go to *aamc.org/first/creditscore*.

- There's an abundance of resources to help you through this process—including those provided by your prehealth advisor, the pages that follow in this book, and the AAMC's Financial Information, Resources, Services, and Tools (FIRST) program. FIRST provides a wide range of resources to help medical school applicants and students make smart decisions about student loans, effectively manage their education debt, and expand their financial skills. The AAMC also provides financial management assistance through a free financial literacy program called SALT. SALT provides practical information on budgeting, money management, credit, debt management, and more. Sign up for your free SALT account at *saltmoney.org/AAMCpremed*.

- The financial aid package offered by each medical school may be a significant factor when you're deciding which offer to accept. For information on this and other considerations, see Chapter 6, "Choosing the Schools That Are Right for You."

3. Maintain Good Credit

- Some medical schools require a credit history as part of the financial aid application and require that applicants resolve any credit problems before they matriculate. Some medical schools will grant a delay of matriculation to an accepted applicant who must address credit problems. Applicants are advised to contact financial aid offices at the medical schools they're interested in to discuss financial aid eligibility and, if necessary, resolve any outstanding credit problems.

Tips to Help Your Credit Score

- Pay your bills on time.

- Limit your credit accounts.

- Keep balances below your credit limit and pay off debt.

- Pay down debt whenever possible. If you can't pay off the debt, at least pay more than the minimum amount due.

- Stay current on all outstanding credit obligations.

- Check your credit report regularly at *annualcreditreport.com*.

Types of Financial Aid

How Will You Pay for Medical School?

First, remember that you're not alone. While the ultimate financial responsibility for your medical education rests with you and your family, there are many resources and tools to help you. The financial aid officer at your medical school will assist you, but you'll also want to talk to your prehealth advisor and familiarize yourself with the Financial Aid Fact Sheets from the AAMC's FIRST program (*aamc.org/first*). Examples of additional financial resources from FIRST include the Debt, Costs, and Loan Repayment Fact Card (Figure 10.2) and information on student loans (Table 10.2).

Figure 10.2. Medical Student Education: Debt, Costs, and Loan Repayment Fact Card.

October 2017 — AAMC

Medical Student Education: Debt, Costs, and Loan Repayment Fact Card

Class of 2017	Public	Private	All
Pct. with Ed. Debt	77%	72%	75%
Mean (indebted only)	$181,179 (↑0%)	$206,204 (↑1%)	$190,694 (↑1%)
Median (indebted only)	$180,000 (↑0%)	$202,000 (↑1%)	$192,000 (↑1%)

Education Debt (including premed) of:	Public	Private	All
$100,000 or more	82%	83%	83%
$200,000 or more	43%	57%	48%
$300,000 or more	10%	21%	14%
Planning to enter loan forgiveness/repayment program:			46%

Education Debt Breakdown	% Graduates	Median
Premedical Education Debt	32%	$25,000
Medical Education Debt	72%	$180,000

Non-Education Debt	% Graduates	Median
Credit Cards	14%	$5,000
Residency/Relocation Loans	3%	$12,000

Source: FIRST analysis of AAMC 2017 GQ data. Education debt figures include premedical education debt plus medical education debt. Non-education debt collected by category.

Cost, M1 In-State, 2017-18	Public	Private
Median Tuition & Fees	$36,937 (↑1%)	$59,605 (↑4%)
Median Cost of Attendance (COA)	$60,945 (↑3%)	$82,278 (↑2%)
Median 4-Yr. COA for Class of 2018	$243,902 (↑1%)	$322,767 (↑3%)

Source: AAMC TSF Survey data from 88 public schools and 54 private schools.

aamc.org/FIRST

Sample Repayment – $192,000 in Federal Direct Loans

Description	Repayment Years	Monthly Payment	Interest Cost	Total Repayment
PAYE during residency and after with $185,000 starting salary	Residency: 3 Post-Res.: 17	$310 to $360 $1,500 to $2,200	$244,000	$390,000 then ~$46,000 forgiven
REPAYE during residency and after with $185,000 starting salary	Residency: 3 Post-Res.: 18	$310 to $360 $1,500 to $2,300	$213,000	$405,000
REPAYE during residency and after with $250,000 starting salary	Residency: 4 Post-Res.: 12	$310 to $380 $2,200 to $2,800	$160,000	$352,000
Forbearance during residency, then Standard	Residency: 3 Post-Res.: 10	$0 $2,900	$156,000	$348,000
Forbearance during residency, then Standard	Residency: 7 Post-Res.: 10	$0 $3,500	$226,000	$418,000
REPAYE during residency and after with $140,000 starting salary and PSLF	Residency: 3 Post-Res.: 7	$310 to $360 $1,100 to $1,300	$113,000	$113,000 then remaining balance forgiven

Notes: PAYE is Pay As You Earn. REPAYE is Revised Pay As You Earn. PSLF is the federal Public Service Loan Forgiveness program. All figures are approximate, rounded for clarity, and estimated for a 2018 graduate. Full assumptions for each scenario available on request. Salaries in 2016 dollars. Non-PSLF amounts forgiven are taxable.

2017 1st Post-MD Year estimated median stipend: $54,600
Federal PAYE/REPAYE monthly payment based on above stipend: $300
See aamc.org/stloan for state and federal loan repayment/scholarship programs.

Interest Rates for federal Graduate/Professional loans disbursed 7/1/17 to 6/30/18
Direct Unsubsidized: 6.00%   Direct PLUS: 7.00%   Rates change annually

Contact Information
Julie Fresne, jfresne@aamc.org
Jay Youngclaus, jy@aamc.org
Matthew Shick, mshick@aamc.org
Joe Bañez, jbanez@aamc.org

The AAMC is the leading source of education debt management information for medical students and residents including the MedLoans® Organizer and Calculator.

aamc.org/FIRST

Table 10.2. Federal Student Loans for Medical Students

Characteristics	Direct Unsubsidized Loan	Direct PLUS Loan	Loans for Disadvantaged Students	Primary Care Loan
Lender	The federal government	The federal government	Medical school financial aid office on behalf of the Department of HHS	Medical school financial aid office on behalf of the Department of HHS
Based on Need	No	No	Yes[1]	Yes[2]
Citizenship Requirement	U.S. citizen, U.S. national, or U.S. permanent resident	U.S. citizen, U.S. national, or U.S. permanent resident	U.S. citizen, U.S. national, or U.S. permanent resident	U.S. citizen, U.S. national, or U.S. permanent resident
Borrowing Limits	$40,500–$47,167/year, $224,000 cumulative maximum for premed and medical borrowing[3]	Annual cost of attendance minus other financial aid	Up to cost of attendance (third- and fourth-year students may receive additional funds to repay previous educational loans received while attending medical school)[3]	Up to cost of attendance (third- and fourth-year students may receive additional funds to repay previous educational loans received while attending medical school)[3]
Interest Rate	For loans disbursed after July 1, 2013, the rate is fixed for the life of the loan. These fixed rates are calculated every July 1st and are effective for loans disbursed during the next academic year. For current rates, visit *studentaid.ed.gov/types/loans/interest-rates.*	For loans disbursed after July 1, 2013, the rate is fixed for the life of the loan. These fixed rates are calculated every July 1st and are effective for loans disbursed during the next academic year. For current rates, visit *studentaid.ed.gov/types/loans/interest-rates.*	5%	5%
Interest Subsidy	No	No	While in school, deferment, and grace period	While in school, deferment, and grace period
Grace Period	6 months	None	1 year	1 year
Deferments	While in school and other possible deferment periods based on eligibility (check your promissory note or ask your financial aid officer)	While in school and 6 months after separating from school (post-enrollment deferment)	While in school and during approved eligible activities	While in school and during a primary care residency (check your promissory note or ask your financial aid officer)
Repayment Requirements	Repayment plans and postponement options exist during residency and beyond	Repayment plans and postponement options exist during residency and beyond	Minimum: $40/month; 10 to 25 years to repay, at the discretion of the institution; may be eligible for federal loan consolidation	Minimum: $40/month; 10 to 25 years to repay; not eligible for loan consolidation
Prepayment Penalties	None			
Allowable Cancellations	Death or total and permanent disability			

1. Parent financial information is required for consideration for dependent students.
2. Borrower must agree upon signing loan agreement to enter and complete a primary care residency and practice in a primary care field, which together must be a total of 10 years in length or until the loan is repaid in full, whichever occurs first. Parent financial information is required for consideration for dependent students.
3. Both annual and aggregate maximums are subject to change, pending congressional action.

Loans

It's likely that your primary financial funding for medical school will come from federal student loans—a form of financial aid. They are normally the first type of loan suggested, before you consider private loans. Table 10.2 provides specific information about four of the most common federal loans used by medical students:

- Direct Unsubsidized Loans

- Direct PLUS Loans

- Loans for Disadvantaged Students (LDS)

- Primary Care Loans (PCL)

Medical school is expensive. However, strong job security and excellent income potential should enable any medical school graduate, practicing in any specialty, to repay education debt and provide for a secure living and retirement.

Grants and Scholarships

When it comes to financing your medical education, the best money is free money, often referred to as "gift aid," which you don't have to repay. While grants and scholarships are likely to cover only a portion of your overall educational costs, it's worth noting that many students get some degree of funding from these sources. The source of gift aid can be from the federal government, the state government, other outside resources, and your medical school. Your medical school financial aid officer is the best source of information about which grants and scholarships may be available to you.

The Financial Aid Application Process

The financial aid process may vary slightly by institution, so you'll want to discuss each school's requirements with the financial aid officer. Generally, most schools require that you're a U.S. citizen or permanent resident, that you're making satisfactory academic progress, and that you're in compliance with Selective Service registration requirements.

Regardless of the medical school, there's a standard process for applying for federal financial aid.

Step 1. Fill Out the FAFSA

Completing the Free Application for Federal Student Aid (FAFSA) is the first step toward getting federal aid for medical school. Completing the FAFSA online is easy and free. The schools listed on your FAFSA will receive your financial information to then determine your eligibility for aid. Some schools may require parental information; check with the financial aid offices of the schools you're applying to for their requirements.

Step 2. Investigate Other Sources of Aid

Contact the financial aid offices at the medical schools you're interested in to investigate other sources of institutional aid, such as loans, scholarships, and grants.

Step 3. Receive and Reply to the Award Letter

Once your FAFSA and other required forms are received and processed by a medical school's financial aid office, you'll receive an award letter indicating the types and amounts of financial aid you qualify for—along with directions for accepting or declining the aid. Be sure to follow the instructions to receive your financial aid in a timely manner. For more information on award letters, review the What Is an Award Letter? Fact Sheet: *students-residents.aamc.org/financial-aid/article/what-is-an-award-letter*.

When awarding aid, each financial aid office has principles that are guided by multiple factors. The aid package is determined by eligibility for federal aid, available institutional resources, family resources, and the institution's mission. Additionally, the school compares the cost of attendance and other external variables before making a final determination of aid eligibility. For eligibility and additional details, talk with the financial aid officer at the medical school you plan to attend. If you're not sure what to ask, review the Top 10 Questions Premeds Should Ask Medical School Financial Aid Officers at *students-residents.aamc.org/financial-aid/article/top-10-questions-pre-meds-should-ask-medical-school/*.

How Medical Schools Determine Eligibility for Financial Aid

Medical schools are sensitive to the financial needs of students. Guided by federal regulations, the financial aid officer will determine your aid eligibility by examining the following questions.

How Much Does It Cost?

The cost of medical education includes tuition, fees, books, supplies, equipment, and living expenses. These components make up the school's cost of attendance (COA) and vary by school. (You can find out the tuition and fees and COA of each medical school on the Medical School Admission Requirements™ website, *aamc.org/msar*.)

What Are Your Resources?

The next area that will be calculated is the amount you'll be required to pay toward the cost of the education. This amount, called the expected family contribution (EFC), is determined through a need-analysis formula to ensure that all students are treated equitably. Both income and assets are considered.

Even though you're considered independent for purposes of federal loans, many institutions require parental financial information to determine eligibility for institutional grants, scholarships, and school-based loans. School officials use this information to assess the student's ability to pay rather than willingness to pay, helping ensure that certain types of aid are awarded to students with the greatest need.

What Additional Resources Are Needed?

Finally, the financial aid office will subtract your EFC from the institution's total cost of attendance. The remainder determines how much aid you'll need for the upcoming academic year. At this point, the medical school will send you an "award letter" detailing the amount and type of financial aid available to you.

You'll be asked to accept or decline the offer (or a portion of it) and return the letter to the school. (The amount of financial aid an institution offers may be an important factor in choosing which school to attend. Review Chapter 6 for additional information and guidance on making your selection. To further assist you in the analysis of your award letters, all accepted applicants are given complimentary access to the MedLoans Organizer and Calculator at *aamc.org/medloans*. This tool can be used to clearly see the total cost associated with the financing options provided in the award letters.)

Forgiveness and Repayment Assistance Programs

Loan forgiveness and repayment programs are available for students interested in reducing their education loan debt through service. These are great options if your career goals align with those of the particular repayment or forgiveness program. The programs vary in structure, requirements, and award amounts.

The federal government provides both service commitment and loan repayment benefits to medical students interested in pursuing careers in primary care and to those committed to working in medically underserved areas.

Additionally, the federal grovernment has a loan forgiveness program to reward borrowers who choose to work in public service, and borrowers can also take advantage of repayment plans offering loan forgiveness if a balance still remains at the end of their loan term.

Some state programs are available to students and graduates in return for a commitment to serve in the state's areas of need. Review the Loan Repayment/Forgiveness and Scholarship Programs database at *aamc.org/stloan*.

The U.S. Armed Forces have programs that offer support to students enrolled in civilian medical schools in exchange for service in the branch that provided the funding.

Federal Loans and Repayment

The benefits available with the federal student loan programs include these:

For additional details on service commitment and loan forgiveness, please review the Repayment Assistance Through Forgiveness, Scholarships, or Service Fact Sheet at *aamc.org/repayasst*.

- **Peace of mind.** Payments are not required until after medical school is over. Payments can even be postponed throughout residency, if a borrower doesn't want to make payments during that time.

- **Fixed interest rates.** Rates will not rise (once the loan has been disbursed), and interest rate reductions may even be available if borrowers elect automatic electronic payment and/or make their payments on time.

- **Various repayment plans.** Flexible plans are available to make payments affordable— even during residency.

- **Education tax credits or deductions.** Some borrowers may be eligible for tax benefits; consult Publication 970 from the IRS for more information (*irs.gov/pub/irs-pdf/p970.pdf*).

As you near graduation, your financial aid office and your loan servicers will supply the details you need to successfully manage your debt after graduation.

A Final Word About Financing Your Medical Education

The AAMC has a variety of financial information, resources, services, and tools for students and residents interested in learning about debt management. For help with accomplishing your financial goals and understanding your options for paying for medical school, review FIRST's Financial Aid Fact Sheets, watch a video, or sign up to participate in a live webinar at *aamc.org/first*.

Service Commitment and Loan Forgiveness Programs

Learn more about these programs at the websites listed below, and review FIRST's Consumer and Federal Financial Aid Resources webpage at *students-residents.aamc.org/financial-aid/article/resources*:

AAMC Loan Repayment/Forgiveness Scholarship Programs Database: *aamc.org/stloan*

Indian Health Services (IHS): *ihs.gov/careeropps/loanrepayment/*

National Health Service Corps: *nhsc.hrsa.gov/index.html*

NIH Loan Repayment: *www.lrp.nih.gov/index.aspx*

Public Service Loan Forgiveness (PSLF): *studentaid.ed.gov/sa/repay-loans/forgiveness-cancellation/public-service*

U.S. Air Force: *airforce.com/education*

U.S. Army: *goarmy.com/amedd/hpsp.html*

U.S. Navy: *navy.com/careers/healthcare/physicians/*

 Worksheets at the end of chapters in this guide are available in fillable PDF format at *aamc.org/msar-resources*.

MONTHLY INCOME:

Financial aid   _____

Investment income   _____

Gifts   _____

Other   _____

Total Fixed Income   _____

MONTHLY FIXED EXPENSES:

Tuition and fees   _____

Books and supplies   _____

Regular savings   _____

Rent/mortgage   _____

Phone   _____

Taxes (federal, state)   _____

Vehicle payments   _____

Other transportation   _____

Personal loans   _____

Education loans   _____

Insurance (life and health)   _____

Home/renter insurance   _____

Auto insurance   _____

Auto registration/taxes   _____

Other   _____

Total Fixed Expenses   _____

MONTHLY VARIABLE EXPENSES:

Food/household supplies   _____

Dining out   _____

Clothes   _____

Laundry/dry cleaning   _____

Gas, oil, auto maintenance   _____

Parking   _____

Medical/dental/eye care   _____

Entertainment   _____

Travel/vacation   _____

Utilities   _____

CDs/books/journals   _____

Personal care   _____

Subscriptions   _____

Cable TV and internet   _____

Credit card payments   _____

Charity/contributions/gifts   _____

Savings for interviews/relocation   _____

Test prep course/materials   _____

Exam/licensing fees   _____

Other   _____

Total Variable Expenses   _____

Plus Total Fixed Expenses   _____

Equals Total Monthly Expenses   _____

Total Income   _____

Less Total Expenses   _____

Equals Total Discretionary Income (or Deficit)   _____

CHAPTER 11

Baccalaureate-MD Programs

> Throughout high school, I pursued many opportunities related to my passion for medicine. When I began my senior year, I wanted to convert this passion into a lifelong career, but I wasn't sure how. When I came across baccalaureate-MD (BS-MD) programs while searching the web for possible premed courses I could take, I was immediately attracted to the many advantages they typically provide: automatic acceptance into medical school, no required major, early clinical exposure, and the potential to save money in application costs.
>
> When researching programs, be sure to look at the school's mission and application requirements and the number of years required to earn the BS-MD degree, as they all differ. Start early, make a list of programs that you are interested in, and be sure to seek out assistance from your guidance counselor. There is also a wealth of information available online and from the AAMC.
>
> With their accelerated course schedules and various required commitments, BS-MD programs may not be for everyone. Remember to ask yourself whether this is the best path for you before starting the application process. If your answer is yes, the list of BS-MD programs in this chapter will help you achieve your dreams of becoming a physician. My experiences with being part of a BS-MD program have been nothing less than excellent. I have had the opportunity to meet and interact with a multitude of medical students and physician mentors while also gaining an extensive amount of clinical experience all as a college student. I'm confident that my enriched undergraduate education has provided me with a solid foundation to be successful in medical school and as a future physician for my patients.

Anisha Guda
Senior, FAME BS-MD Candidate
University of Texas Health Science Center
at San Antonio Long School of Medicine
Class of 2018, BS
Class of 2021, MD

According to the AAMC's 2017 Graduation Questionnaire (GQ), about 91% of students focus on obtaining their undergraduate degree before earning their MD, about 2.7% graduate from joint baccalaureate-MD programs, and 3.1% earn a joint MD-PhD.

Purposes of Baccalaureate-MD Programs

The purposes of these programs vary by institution and may include the following:

- To permit highly qualified students to plan and complete a broad liberal arts education before starting their medical studies

- To admit highly qualified students with the desired combination of experiences, attributes, and metrics who have demonstrated an early commitment to medicine and whose goals align with the mission of the medical school

- To enhance diversity in the premedical and medical education environments

- To reduce the total number of years required to complete the MD degree

- To educate physicians likely to practice in particular geographic areas or work with medically underserved populations

- To reduce the costs of a medical education

- To prepare physician-scientists and future leaders in health policy

Potential applicants should familiarize themselves with the mission, statement of goals, and requirements of each combined-degree program in which they have an interest to ensure an appropriate match between their educational and professional goals and those of the program. This information can usually be found on the medical school's website.

These programs typically represent relationships between a medical school and one or more undergraduate colleges located in the same geographic region. They can be a part of the same university system, or they can span different institutions. Learning about the schools involved in a baccalaureate-MD program can help you better understand the program's mission and features.

Admission is open to highly qualified, mature students at the high school or early college level who are committed to a future career in medicine. Admitted students tend to have a set of life experiences that signal their maturity and commitment. For more information, see the Medical School Admission Requirements™ website, specifically the About section for baccalaureate-MD programs (*aamc.org/msar*). State-supported schools generally admit few out-of-state applicants to their baccalaureate-MD programs; private schools tend to have greater flexibility about state of residency.

While academic requirements vary among the schools sponsoring these programs, they typically include successful completion of prerequisite courses in biology, chemistry, physics, English, mathematics, and social science courses as well as a minimum grade point average and standardized test scores. Calculus and foreign-language courses are also frequently required; a computer science course is sometimes recommended. Admission to the MD portion of the program may occur immediately or after a student completes a prescribed number of semesters with a minimum grade point average (GPA). In some programs, students are not required to take the MCAT exam; in other programs, a minimum MCAT score must be attained to progress through the program.

Progressing through the program from the undergraduate to the medical curricula is usually contingent on a student's achieving specific criteria in terms of standardized test scores, GPAs, and meeting the school's expectations for personal and professional behavior.

If you're interested in a combined baccalaureate-MD program, you should consult your school counselor to ensure that you're enrolled in a curriculum that incorporates the courses required for admission to the program and readies you for the premedical phase of this pathway. The requirements may involve specific high school or college courses. If you're a college freshman or sophomore interested in these programs, please speak with your school's prehealth advisor. For additional information about specific programs, contact each school directly.

This chapter contains lists of combined baccalaureate-MD programs by state and by number of years to complete them. For information about the programs, see the Medical School Admission Requirements website.

How to Find and Prepare for Baccalaureate-MD Programs

Baccalaureate-MD programs can be a great option for high school seniors. If you're a high school student, talk with your school counselor about the programs that may be a good option for you. You can use the Medical School Admission Requirements website to search for medical schools with baccalaureate-MD programs. Also, explore opportunities at your school or in your community to get engaged in health care issues and shadow health care professionals. These experiences will help you understand how you fit within a career in medicine and perhaps even the kind of medical setting that suits your interests, aptitudes, goals, and personality.

Each year, new programs are being developed, and many are aimed toward creating an option for students who are traditionally unrepresented in medicine. In Chapter 4, you can read more about diversity initiatives in medicine, and in Chapter 7, you can find more information about the holistic review of candidates who apply to medical school. With this in mind, you can use the worksheet at the end of this chapter to evaluate the mission statements of the programs that you are interested in and decide which ones may be a good fit for you.

Medical Schools Offering Combined Baccalaureate-MD Programs, by State, 2017–2018

ALABAMA

University of Alabama School of Medicine–Birmingham

University of South Alabama College of Medicine

CALIFORNIA

California Northstate University College of Medicine

University of California, Riverside, School of Medicine

COLORADO

University of Colorado School of Medicine

CONNECTICUT

University of Connecticut School of Medicine

DISTRICT OF COLUMBIA

George Washington University School of Medicine and Health Sciences

Howard University College of Medicine

FLORIDA

Charles E. Schmidt College of Medicine at Florida Atlantic University

University of Central Florida College of Medicine

University of Florida College of Medicine

University of Miami Leonard M. Miller School of Medicine

USF Health Morsani College of Medicine

GEORGIA

Medical College of Georgia at Augusta University

ILLINOIS

Northwestern University The Feinberg School of Medicine

University of Chicago Division of the Biological Sciences The Pritzker School of Medicine

University of Illinois College of Medicine

MASSACHUSETTS

Boston University School of Medicine

MICHIGAN

Wayne State University School of Medicine

MINNESOTA

University of Minnesota Medical School

MISSOURI

Saint Louis University School of Medicine

University of Missouri–Kansas City School of Medicine

Washington University School of Medicine in St. Louis

NEVADA

University of Nevada, Reno School of Medicine

NEW JERSEY

Cooper Medical School of Rowan University

Rutgers, New Jersey Medical School

Rutgers, Robert Wood Johnson Medical School

NEW MEXICO

University of New Mexico School of Medicine

NEW YORK

Albany Medical College

CUNY School of Medicine

Hofstra Northwell School of Medicine at Hofstra University

State University of New York Downstate Medical Center College of Medicine

State University of New York Upstate Medical University

Stony Brook University School of Medicine

University of Rochester School of Medicine and Dentistry

OHIO

Case Western Reserve University School of Medicine

Northeast Ohio Medical University

University of Cincinnati College of Medicine

The University of Toledo College of Medicine

PENNSYLVANIA

Drexel University College of Medicine

Lewis Katz School of Medicine at Temple University

Sidney Kimmel Medical College at Thomas Jefferson University

PUERTO RICO

Ponce Health Sciences University School of Medicine

RHODE ISLAND

The Warren Alpert Medical School of Brown University

SOUTH CAROLINA

University of South Carolina School of Medicine

TENNESSEE

Meharry Medical College

TEXAS

Baylor College of Medicine

University of Texas Health Science Center at San Antonio Long School of Medicine

University of Texas Rio Grande Valley School of Medicine

VIRGINIA

Eastern Virginia Medical School

Virginia Commonwealth University School of Medicine

Medical Schools Offering Combined Baccalaureate-MD Programs, by Number of Years, 2017–2018

6 YEARS

University of Missouri–Kansas City School of Medicine

6–7 YEARS

California Northstate University College of Medicine

Northeast Ohio Medical University

Sidney Kimmel Medical College at Jefferson University

University of Miami Leonard M. Miller School of Medicine

7 YEARS

Albany Medical College

Boston University School of Medicine (8-year option available)

Cooper Medical School of Rowan University

CUNY School of Medicine

Drexel University College of Medicine

George Washington University School of Medicine and Health Sciences

Meharry Medical College

Northeast Ohio Medical University

Northwestern University The Feinberg School of Medicine

Rutgers, New Jersey Medical School

Rutgers, Robert Wood Johnson Medical School

University of Florida College of Medicine

University of Illinois College of Medicine

University of Minnesota Medical School

University of Nevada, Reno School of Medicine

University of South Carolina School of Medicine

University of Texas Health Science Center at San Antonio Long School of Medicine

8 YEARS

Albany Medical College

Baylor College of Medicine

Case Western Reserve University School of Medicine

Charles E. Schmidt College of Medicine at Florida Atlantic University

Eastern Virginia Medical School

George Washington University School of Medicine and Health Sciences

Hofstra Northwell School of Medicine at Hofstra University

Howard University College of Medicine

Keck School of Medicine of the University of Southern California

Northeast Ohio Medical University

Rutgers, New Jersey Medical School

Rutgers, Robert Wood Johnson Medical School

Saint Louis University School of Medicine

State University of New York Upstate Medical University

Stony Brook University School of Medicine

University of Alabama School of Medicine

University of California, San Diego, School of Medicine

University of Cincinnati College of Medicine

University of Colorado School of Medicine

University of Connecticut School of Medicine

University of New Mexico School of Medicine

University of Rochester School of Medicine and Dentistry

University of South Alabama College of Medicine

Virginia Commonwealth University School of Medicine

The Warren Alpert Medical School of Brown University

Wayne State University School of Medicine

9 YEARS

University of Cincinnati College of Medicine

Worksheets at the end of chapters in this guide are available in fillable PDF format at *aamc.org/msar-resources*.

1. **Name of Baccalaureate-MD Program** _____

What is the mission of this program? _____

Why are you interested in this program? _____

# of Years: _____   Accepts out-of-state? _____   Application deadline: _____

When eligible to apply: College freshman ____   High school senior ____   Other _____

2. **Name of Baccalaureate-MD Program** _____

What is the mission of this program? _____

Why are you interested in this program? _____

# of Years: _____   Accepts out-of-state? _____   Application deadline: _____

When eligible to apply: College freshman ____   High school senior ____   Other _____

3. **Name of Baccalaureate-MD Program** _____

What is the mission of this program? _____

Why are you interested in this program? _____

# of Years: _____   Accepts out-of-state? _____   Application deadline: _____

When eligible to apply: College freshman ____   High school senior ____   Other _____

4. **Name of Baccalaureate-MD Program** _____

What is the mission of this program? _____

Why are you interested in this program? _____

# of Years: _____   Accepts out-of-state? _____   Application deadline: _____

When eligible to apply: College freshman ____   High school senior ____   Other _____

CHAPTER 12

MD-PhD Programs

> *Volunteering in a free health clinic was the first time I realized I wanted to become a doctor. It was striking to see how an illness could completely upend a person's circumstances, allowing physicians the opportunity to use their expertise to have an extraordinary impact on a life. Moreover, I was fascinated by the process of correlating a patient's symptoms with the pathophysiology of disease. I knew then that medicine would be a meaningful and gratifying application of my love for science.*
>
> *At the time, I was also conducting basic science research. A curious person by nature, I wanted to know why and how things work. Research not only enabled me to explore my hypotheses, but also allowed me to engage in the scientific community. Together with the advances being made by passionate scientists worldwide, I wanted my research to help answer the many questions remaining in medicine.*
>
> *I chose to pursue an MD-PhD program because I wanted to have an immediate impact on patients' lives while advancing our knowledge of health and disease through research. As a physician-scientist, I will have a unique opportunity to have scientific knowledge inform my work at the bedside and have my clinical work guide and energize my research. Ultimately, I aspire to applying the rigorous clinical and scientific training afforded by the MD-PhD program to help both individuals and populations afflicted by disease.*

Janice L. Farlow
MD-PhD Candidate
Indiana University
School of Medicine
Class of 2017

The Education of a Physician-Scientist

Although about 91% of students entering medical school each year choose to study in MD-only programs, about 9% enter into joint degree programs: 3% enroll in MD-PhD programs, 3% enroll in BA- or BS-MD programs, and 3% enroll in other joint degree programs (e.g., MD-MPH, MD-MS).

Physician-scientists—those who are trained in both medicine and research—are greatly needed in today's world. There is a synergy that results when experimental thinking and clinical practice are joined, and that combination is found among those who have completed both MD and PhD programs. These individuals help translate the achievements of basic research into active clinical practice and, in doing so, strengthen the link between medical knowledge and research as they study, prevent, diagnose, and treat disease. If this is the path you prefer, you'll enjoy a busy, challenging, and rewarding career.

Advantages of the MD-PhD Dual Degree

One route to a career as a physician-scientist is enrollment in a combined MD-PhD program. Although you can complete a PhD program before or after receiving your MD degree, there are several advantages to pursuing joint MD-PhD education:

- The greatest advantage of the dual-degree program is the integration of research and clinical training. This integrated approach may include training opportunities that cross departments and interactions with teams composed of both basic scientists and clinical investigators.

- You can save a significant amount of time. Most MD-PhD programs can be completed in seven or eight years, compared with the nine or more years it would take to earn both degrees independently.

- Students in MD-PhD programs have access to opportunities for research and faculty mentoring to an extent frequently unavailable to MD-only students. As a result, these students are often able to enhance their mastery of the basic science needed to identify patients' underlying clinical problems and, ultimately, use that information to develop improvements in diagnosis and treatment. To learn more about available programs and how to apply, go to *aamc.org/mdphd*.

Paths to a Research Career

If you're interested in a career in research but you aren't sure whether you want to pursue a dual MD-PhD degree, here are some other options you can explore:

- **PhD in biomedical sciences.** You can earn a PhD in biomedical sciences in graduate programs at medical schools. Such programs typically include one or two years of core coursework, lab rotations to help you select a mentor in your chosen field of research, and three to four years of doctoral research. To learn more about available programs and how to apply, go to *aamc.org/phd*.

> ### Professional School Fair—MD-PhD: Is It Right for Me?
>
> In this videocast, the leaders of medical school MD-PhD programs describe undergraduate preparation and application processes and discuss training in MD-PhD programs and postgraduate career opportunities: *videocast.nih.gov/Summary. asp?File=15209&bhcp=1.*

- **MS degree or PhD in clinical investigation.** You might also consider graduate work leading to a master's degree or PhD in clinical investigation. These programs, which you can pursue jointly or after receiving your MD degree, are offered at many medical schools and biomedical graduate schools throughout the country.

- **Year-enrichment program.** Another option is to take a year away from your MD program to conduct research under the direction of a mentor in a scholars program. Three such programs are the **Fogarty International Clinical Research Scholarship Program**, the **National Institutes of Health (NIH) Medical Research Scholars Program**, and the **Howard Hughes Medical Institute (HHMI) Research Fellows Program**. For details, see *fogartyscholars.org*, *cc.nih.gov/training/mrsp*, and *hhmi.org/grants/individuals/medical-fellows*. In addition, many medical schools offer similar opportunities for their students.

Research Specialties

Like their PhD-only counterparts, people who hold a combined degree can pursue many scientific specialties. Most students earn their PhDs in biomedical disciplines such as biochemistry, biomedical engineering, biophysics, cell biology, genetics, immunology, microbiology, neuroscience, and pharmacology.

It's important to know, however, that not every research specialty is offered at every medical school and that curricula can vary from institution to institution. In some schools, for example, MD-PhD students complete their graduate work in the social sciences or humanities—fields of study outside laboratory disciplines—in areas such as anthropology, computational biology, economics, engineering, health care policy, mathematics, physics, and sociology.

To learn more, go to *students-residents.aamc.org/choosing-medical-career/article/md-phd-social-sciences-or-humanities-it-right-me*.

View a summary of MD-PhD programs and graduate fields of study at *aamc-orange.global.ssl.fastly.net/production/media/filer_public/74/a1/74a1d614-58a0-4acf-862a-ec6f54081713/individual_md-phd_program_info_prospective_applicants_table_092116.pdf*.

Clinical Specialties

MD-PhD students can pursue any of many clinical specialties. The clinical specialty choices of students graduating from MD-PhD programs over the past five years indicate strong interest in internal medicine, pathology, and pediatrics.

Compared with MD-only graduates, MD-PhD graduates are more likely to enter residencies in radiation oncology, child neurology, and pathology and less likely to go into family medicine, emergency medicine, and obstetrics/gynecology. The majority of dual-degree students enter research residency programs after graduation. A very small percentage of program graduates choose not to enter clinical residency and go straight into a research postdoctoral fellowship training.

The Typical Program

Almost all U.S. and Canadian medical schools have MD-PhD programs in one or more areas of specialization. (You can find a listing of MD-PhD programs available at AAMC member medical schools at *aamc.org/individual-md-phd-program-info-2016*.) Some programs are relatively small, with a total of a dozen or so students over eight years of training (one or two new students each year), and others are much larger, with a total enrollment of around 190 (up to 24 new students enrolled annually). The total number of matriculants in 2017 was 649, with 44% women and 56% men. You can find Table B-8: U.S. Medical School MD-PhD Applications and Matriculants by School, In-State Status, and Sex, 2017–2018 at *aamc.org/download/321544/data/factstableb8.pdf*.

Although there are differences among programs, core elements are common to almost all. The typical program is completed in seven to eight years and includes the following:

- Completion of the first two years of combined medical and graduate school coursework

- Three to five years of doctoral research, including the completion of a thesis project

- A return to medical school for core clinical training and electives during the final years of the medical curriculum

At most schools, integrated approaches to graduate and medical education have been introduced throughout the curriculum, quite extensively in some programs. In addition, most programs engage students in a wide range of other activities to enrich their training experience. Many MD-PhD programs, in addition to a PhD in traditional biomedical sciences, offer graduate training in social sciences and humanities. For a full list of these opportunities, go to *students-residents.aamc.org/choosing-medical-career/article/md-phd-social-sciences-or-humanities-it-right-me*.

Residency Programs After Graduation

After medical school, most MD-PhD students transition to residencies just like a traditional medical student. A number of residency programs around the country offer highly structured programs in which research is fully integrated into clinical training. They differ in their overall composition but generally offer a shortened residency training period. For more information, visit *students-residents.aamc.org/choosing-medical-career/article/career-paths-md-phd-graduates*.

Application and Admission

Nearly all MD-PhD programs participate in the American Medical College Application Service® (AMCAS®), described in Chapter 7.

If you choose to pursue the dual-degree program, you'll designate yourself as a combined MD-PhD training applicant and complete two additional essays: one explaining why you are interested in the joint training program and the other describing your research experience. Specifics in the application process—and the prerequisites required for admission—vary from school to school. (Some institutions, for example, require GRE scores.) For complete information about a dual-degree program that interests you, review the program description at the appropriate medical school's website.

Where Physician-Scientists Work

About 75% of MD-PhD graduates are employed as faculty members in academic medical centers or in pharmaceutical companies. Other graduates work in a wide range of other capacities, including as scientists in biotechnology firms, the federal government, clinical medicine, and basic research.

Source: LF Brass, et al. Are MD-PhD programs meeting their goals? An analysis of career choices made by graduates of 24 MD-PhD programs. Academic Medicine 2010; 85(4):692–701.

Factors Considered by Admissions Committees

Admissions committee members will review the application materials for the usual experiences, attributes, and metrics that are important for admitting students to MD-only programs (see Chapter 8). But because MD-PhD applicants plan to become both physicians and scientists, committee members will also look for evidence of an applicant's passion and aptitude for research. They accomplish this largely through reviewing the applicant's personal statement, which includes a description of research experiences, and letters of evaluation from faculty or researchers with whom the applicant has worked. In particular, committee members seek confirmation of the following:

- Relevant and substantive research experience during or after college

- An appreciation for and understanding of the work of physician-scientists

- Intellectual drive, research ability, and perseverance

If you hope to pursue the MD-PhD joint degree, you'll be expected to have clinical experience—through volunteer work, shadowing a physician-scientist, or specific training. Other experiences that admissions committee members look for are similar to those of the MD-only candidate: leadership positions, community service activities, and teaching roles.

Finally, it's important to be aware that although significant weight is placed on an applicant's interest and experience in research activities, the applicant is also expected to demonstrate a degree of academic excellence similar to that of people accepted into an MD-only program. For students entering MD-PhD programs in 2017, for example, the mean GPA and total MCAT score were 3.78 and 513.9, respectively (as reported by AMCAS, *aamc.org/download/321548/data/factstableb10.pdf*). Keep in mind, though, that the range of GPAs and MCAT scores for accepted applicants is quite broad in conjunction with other selection criteria.

Acceptance Policies

Just as application requirements vary from school to school, so do acceptance policies. Some institutions permit an applicant who is not accepted to the MD-PhD dual-degree program to pursue admission to the MD-only curriculum. Other medical schools will accept applications from MD-PhD candidates only for both degree programs, and failure to gain admittance to one program precludes consideration from another. Because school policies differ, applicants should clarify these matters with individual schools before applying and let admissions office staff know of their interest in pursuing an MD-only program (if that is the case) should they not be admitted to the dual-degree program.

Financing MD-PhD Programs

The sources of funding for MD-PhD programs vary from school to school. Many schools offer full support for both the MD and PhD components of their education, including tuition waivers, stipends, and health insurance. At other institutions, different degrees of support are available, sometimes only for the PhD component of the program. Before applying to an MD-PhD dual-degree program, you should check with individual programs about the level of financial assistance available.

A significant amount of funding comes from institutional sources and both individual and institutional grants. The latter include the Medical Scientist Training Program (MSTP) sponsored by the National Institutes of Health (NIH), as well as other NIH grants. The MSTP currently has 47 participating programs with a total of 900 trainees. For more information, go to *nigms.nih.gov/Training/InstPredoc/Pages/PredocOverview-MSTP.aspx*. To review the list of medical schools participating in the MSTP, visit *nigms.nih.gov/Training/InstPredoc/Pages/ PredocInst-MSTP.aspx*. You may also want to contact the program officials at the institutions of interest and review the schools' websites for complete information.

Bear in mind that although most MD-PhD programs offer support for their students, additional resources are available. Most take the form of competitive applications submitted by the trainee and a research mentor. They include fellowships from both private sources and a number of NIH institutes. You can review the list of these opportunities at *students-residents.aamc.org/choosing-medical-career/article/financing-your-graduate-education*.

Gap Year and Career Changers

If you have a significant break between earning your bachelor's degree and applying to medical school, you should use some of that time to gain more research and medically related experience (such as working, shadowing, or volunteering in hospitals and clinics). This will help make you a competitive applicant— you can draw on that experience as you complete your medical school applications and interviews. For more information about gaining research experience, see the Aspiring Docs® fact sheet called How to Get Lab Experience, *students-residents.aamc.org/applying-medical-school/article/how-get-lab-experience*.

Additional Information

For additional information and guidance about application to and enrollment in combined MD-PhD programs, please visit the AAMC's website on dual-degree programs at *aamc.org/mdphd* and contact your prehealth advisor and the MD-PhD program director at the medical schools of interest.

Want to learn more? You can find answers to questions frequently asked by students at *students-residents. aamc.org/choosing-medical-career/faq/faq-about-md-phd-programs-and-careers*.

For additional information about MD-PhD programs, see:

Brass LF, Akabas MH, Burnley LD, Engman DM, Wiley CA, Andersen OS. Are MD-PhD programs meeting their goals? An analysis of career choices made by graduates of 24 MD-PhD programs. *Academic Medicine*. 2010;85(4):692–701.

Paik JC, Howard G, Lorenz RG. Postgraduate choices of graduates from medical scientist training programs, 2004–2008. *JAMA*. 2009;302(12):1271–1273.

> **Worksheets at the end of chapters in this guide are available in fillable PDF format at *aamc.org/msar-resources*.**

MD-PhD Programs to Consider Applying To

When researching your options, view the AAMC's table with information on MD-PhD programs online and fill in the chart below to see if you fit the application criteria and may want to apply to the program (*aamc.org/individual-md-phd-program-info-2016*).

Consider Applying?							
Summer Positions?							
GRE Required?							
Non-U.S. Citizens or Non-State Residents Accepted							
Transfer Students?							
Internal PhD Students?							
Internal MD Students?							
Positions Funded?							
Medical Science Training Program (MSTP) Funded?							
Program Name							

CHAPTER 13

U.S. Medical Schools
Accredited by the Liaison Committee on Medical Education (LCME)

Medical School Admission Requirements™ (MSAR®) Website— Complete U.S. Medical School Profiles

For complete, detailed information about each U.S. medical school, including MCAT® and GPA data, school-specific admission requirements and policies, applicant and acceptee statistics, and side-by-side medical school comparisons, purchase a subscription to the Medical School Admission Requirements. For more information about the Medical School Admission Requirements website, a preview of the site, and a complete list of site features, data, and information, visit *aamc.org/msar*.

U.S. Medical Schools

ALABAMA

University of Alabama School of Medicine

University of South Alabama College of Medicine

ARIZONA

University of Arizona College of Medicine–Phoenix

University of Arizona College of Medicine–Tucson

ARKANSAS

University of Arkansas for Medical Sciences
College of Medicine

CALIFORNIA

California Northstate University College of Medicine

California University of Science and Medicine School
of Medicine

David Geffen School of Medicine at UCLA

Keck School of Medicine of the University of Southern California

Loma Linda University School of Medicine

Stanford University School of Medicine

University of California, Davis, School of Medicine

University of California, Irvine, School of Medicine

University of California, Riverside, School of Medicine

University of California, San Diego, School of Medicine

University of California, San Francisco, School of Medicine

COLORADO

University of Colorado School of Medicine

CONNECTICUT

Frank H. Netter MD School of Medicine at Quinnipiac University

University of Connecticut School of Medicine

Yale School of Medicine

DISTRICT OF COLUMBIA

George Washington University School of Medicine and Health Sciences

Georgetown University School of Medicine

Howard University College of Medicine

FLORIDA

Charles E. Schmidt College of Medicine at Florida Atlantic University

Florida International University Herbert Wertheim College of Medicine

Florida State University College of Medicine

Nova Southeastern University Dr. Kiran C. Patel College of Allopathic Medicine

University of Central Florida College of Medicine

University of Florida College of Medicine

University of Miami Leonard M. Miller School of Medicine

USF Health Morsani College of Medicine

GEORGIA

Emory University School of Medicine

Medical College of Georgia at Augusta University

Mercer University School of Medicine

Morehouse School of Medicine

HAWAII

University of Hawaii, John A. Burns School of Medicine

ILLINOIS

Carle Illinois College of Medicine

Chicago Medical School at Rosalind Franklin University of Medicine and Science

Loyola University Chicago Stritch School of Medicine

Northwestern University Feinberg School of Medicine

Rush Medical College of Rush University Medical Center

Southern Illinois University School of Medicine

University of Chicago Division of the Biological Sciences, The Pritzker School of Medicine

University of Illinois College of Medicine

INDIANA

Indiana University School of Medicine

IOWA

University of Iowa Roy J. and Lucille A. Carver College of Medicine

KANSAS

University of Kansas School of Medicine

KENTUCKY

University of Kentucky College of Medicine

University of Louisville School of Medicine

LOUISIANA

Louisiana State University School of Medicine in Shreveport

Louisiana State University School of Medicine in New Orleans

Tulane University School of Medicine

MARYLAND

Johns Hopkins University School of Medicine

Uniformed Services University of the Health Sciences
F. Edward Hébert School of Medicine

University of Maryland School of Medicine

MASSACHUSETTS

Boston University School of Medicine

Harvard Medical School

Tufts University School of Medicine

University of Massachusetts Medical School

MICHIGAN

Central Michigan University College of Medicine

Michigan State University College of
Human Medicine

Oakland University William Beaumont
School of Medicine

University of Michigan Medical School

Wayne State University School of Medicine

Western Michigan University Homer Stryker M.D.
School of Medicine

MINNESOTA

Mayo Medical School

University of Minnesota Medical School

MISSISSIPPI

University of Mississippi School of Medicine

MISSOURI

Saint Louis University School of Medicine

University of Missouri–Columbia School
of Medicine

University of Missouri–Kansas City School
of Medicine

Washington University School of Medicine
in St. Louis

NEBRASKA

Creighton University School of Medicine

University of Nebraska Medical Center
College of Medicine

NEVADA

University of Nevada, Reno School of Medicine

University of Nevada, Las Vegas School of Medicine

NEW HAMPSHIRE

Geisel School of Medicine at Dartmouth

NEW JERSEY

Cooper Medical School of Rowan University

Rutgers, New Jersey Medical School

Rutgers, Robert Wood Johnson Medical School

Seton Hall-Hackensack Meridian School of Medicine

NEW MEXICO

University of New Mexico School of Medicine

NEW YORK

Albany Medical College

Albert Einstein College of Medicine

City University of New York School of Medicine

Columbia University Vagelos College of Physicians
and Surgeons

Donald and Barbara Zucker School of Medicine
at Hofstra/Northwell

Icahn School of Medicine at Mount Sinai

New York Medical College

Jacobs School of Medicine and Biomedical Sciences
at the University at Buffalo

New York University School of Medicine

State University of New York Downstate Medical
Center College of Medicine

State University of New York Upstate
Medical University

Stony Brook University School of Medicine

University of Rochester School of Medicine
and Dentistry

Weill Cornell Medicine

NORTH CAROLINA

The Brody School of Medicine
at East Carolina University

Duke University School of Medicine

University of North Carolina at Chapel Hill
School of Medicine

Wake Forest University School of Medicine
of Wake Forest Baptist Medical Center

NORTH DAKOTA

University of North Dakota School of Medicine
and Health Sciences

OHIO

Case Western Reserve University School of Medicine

Northeast Ohio Medical University

Ohio State University College of Medicine

University of Cincinnati College of Medicine

The University of Toledo College of Medicine

Wright State University Boonshoft School
of Medicine

OKLAHOMA

University of Oklahoma College of Medicine

OREGON

Oregon Health & Science University School
of Medicine

PENNSYLVANIA

Drexel University College of Medicine

Geisinger Commonwealth School of Medicine

Lewis Katz School of Medicine at Temple University

Pennsylvania State University College of Medicine

Perelman School of Medicine at the University
of Pennsylvania

Sidney Kimmel Medical College at Thomas
Jefferson University

University of Pittsburgh School of Medicine

PUERTO RICO

Ponce Health Sciences University School of Medicine

San Juan Bautista School of Medicine

Universidad Central del Caribe School of Medicine

University of Puerto Rico School of Medicine

RHODE ISLAND

The Warren Alpert Medical School
of Brown University

SOUTH CAROLINA

Medical University of South Carolina
College of Medicine

University of South Carolina School of Medicine

University of South Carolina School of Medicine–
Greenville

SOUTH DAKOTA

Sanford School of Medicine, University
of South Dakota

TENNESSEE

East Tennessee State University James H. Quillen
College of Medicine

Meharry Medical College

University of Tennessee Health Science Center
College of Medicine

Vanderbilt University School of Medicine

TEXAS

Baylor College of Medicine

McGovern Medical School at the University
of Texas Health Science Center at Houston

Texas A&M Health Science Center
College of Medicine

Texas Tech University Health Sciences Center
Paul L. Foster School of Medicine

Texas Tech University Health Sciences Center
School of Medicine

University of Texas at Austin Dell Medical School

University of Texas Medical Branch
School of Medicine

University of Texas Health Science Center at San
Antonio Long School of Medicine

University of Texas Rio Grande Valley School
of Medicine

University of Texas Southwestern Medical School

UTAH
University of Utah School of Medicine

VERMONT
University of Vermont Robert Larner, M.D. College of Medicine

VIRGINIA
Eastern Virginia Medical School

University of Virginia School of Medicine

Virginia Commonwealth University School of Medicine

Virginia Tech Carilion School of Medicine

WASHINGTON
University of Washington School of Medicine

Washington State University Elson S. Floyd College of Medicine

WEST VIRGINIA
Marshall University Joan C. Edwards School of Medicine

West Virginia University School of Medicine

Wisconsin
Medical College of Wisconsin

University of Wisconsin School of Medicine and Public Health

CHAPTER 14

Canadian Medical Schools

Accredited by the Liaison Committee on Medical Education (LCME) and by the Committee on Accreditation of Canadian Medical Schools (CACMS)

> *I actually applied broadly to schools in both the United States and Canada. The United States has more than 100 public and private medical schools, whereas Canada has only 17, including 3 that are exclusively French-speaking, and they're all public. However, the curricula in both countries fulfill the same Liaison Committee on Medical Education (LCME) requirements. Canadian medical schools also fulfill the Canadian Committee on Accreditation of Canadian Medical Schools (CACMS) requirements.*
>
> *Ultimately, I decided to enroll in Dalhousie University's medical program, located in my hometown of Halifax, Nova Scotia. Other than the benefit of being home, Dalhousie was particularly attractive to me because of its focus on building clinical skills in students early on. Furthermore, offering smaller class sizes meant that I was able to form strong relationships with my classmates. Those friendships, I knew, would prove key in helping me navigate the thick and thin of what can be a grueling medical education. All Canadian medical schools are affiliated with the Association of American Medical Colleges through the Association of Faculties of Medicine of Canada.*

Henry Annan
MD Candidate
Dalhousie University, Canada
Class of 2018

Selection Criteria

Canadian medical schools vary with respect to the number of years of undergraduate instruction they require of applicants. They also vary in the recommended content covered during premedical undergraduate education. Table 14.1 shows that physics, inorganic and organic chemistry, biology, biochemistry, humanities, and English are the most common required subjects there.

Language of Instruction

Three Canadian medical schools—Laval, Montréal, and Sherbrooke, all located in Quebec province—require students to be fluent in French because all instruction is in that language. Instruction in 13 other schools is in English, and the University of Ottawa offers the MD curriculum in both French and English.

Table 14.1. Subjects Often Required or Recommended by Canadian Medical Schools*

Required or Recommended Subject
Biochemistry
Biology
Biology/Zoology
Calculus
College Mathematics
English
Humanities
Inorganic Chemistry
Organic Chemistry
Physics
Social Sciences

*For specific requirements and recommendations, see the individual school profiles on the Medical School Admission Requirements™ website: aamc.org/msar (subscription required). You can also view coursework requirements on individual medical school websites. Source: AAMC Medical College Admission Requirements website, 2017.

In Canada, universities fall under provincial jurisdiction, and the majority of places in each faculty of medicine are allocated to permanent residents of the province in which the university is located.

Not all faculties of medicine accept applications from international students. Conversely, some faculties of medicine may reserve positions for international students, possibly as part of agreements with foreign governments and institutions. Statistics compiled by the Association of Faculties of Medicine of Canada (*afmc.ca*) show that most medical schools admit international students. In 2016–2017, for example, 108 U.S. students applied to 15 schools, and 1% of those students were accepted, according to the Canadian medical schools that supplied data. In the same year, 277 non-U.S. international students applied to the 15 Canadian medical schools that supplied data, and their success rate was 3%. The success rate for Canadian applicants to the same schools was 19.6%. Additional information about Canadian medical schools can be found in the Association of Faculties of Medicine of Canada 2017 publication of *Admission Requirements of Canadian Faculties of Medicine* (*afmc.ca/publications/admission-requirements-canadian-faculties-medicine*).

Positions filled by international students in Canadian medical schools are not necessarily subsidized by provincial or territorial governments. This means that international students, including U.S. students, may pay higher tuition and fees than Canadian residents.

Academic Record and Suitability

Although an excellent academic record is a very important factor in gaining admission to a Canadian medical school, admissions committees also put a great deal of effort into assessing applicants' suitability for a medical career based on other factors, too. Personal suitability is assessed differently by each school, but in general, personal qualities related to medicine are very important. Applicants who can demonstrate that they possess the qualities considered important in the practice of medicine may sometimes be admitted even if their academic record is not outstanding. Conversely, applicants with outstanding records who don't possess these qualities may not gain a place in medical school.

Most applicants to Canadian medical schools are interviewed before acceptance, so the interview information in Chapter 8 is also relevant for them.

Medical College Admission Test® (MCAT®)

Twelve of the 17 Canadian medical schools require applicants to take the MCAT® exam: Alberta, British Columbia, Calgary, Dalhousie, Manitoba, McGill, McMaster, Memorial, Queen's, Saskatchewan, Toronto, and Western Ontario.

Tuition and Other Compulsory Fees

Because the medical schools in Canada fall under the jurisdiction of provincial governments, annual tuition and compulsory fees vary considerably. Applicants who reside in the province where the medical school is located may pay annual fees ranging from $4,649 to $28,201, with an average of $17,224 (see Table 14.2). Applicants who are Canadian citizens or permanent residents in a different province may pay fees ranging from $9,550 to $28,201, with an average of $19,154, and foreign student applicants can expect to pay fees ranging from $27,966 to $74,962, with an average of $38,837.

Table 14.2. Tuition and Student Fees for 2017–2018 First-Year Students at Canadian Medical Schools (in Canadian Dollars)*

Categories of Students	Range	Average**
In-Province	$4,649–$28,201	$17,224
Canada, Out-of-Province	$9,550–$28,201	$19,154
Visa	$27,966–$74,962	$38,837

*Figures based on data provided in fall 2017.
**Average in-province and out-of-province data were derived from all 17 Canadian schools. Average visa data were derived from six schools that accept foreign students.
Source: The Association of Faculties of Medicine of Canada, 2017.

Other Considerations

Canadian faculties of medicine do not discriminate on the basis of race, religion, or gender in admitting new students. The admission of Aboriginal students (First Nations, Inuit, and Métis) is encouraged at Canadian medical schools, and most allocate positions specifically for Aboriginal applicants, including Laval, Sherbrooke, Montréal, McGill, Ottawa, Queen's, McMaster, Western Ontario, Northern Ontario School of Medicine, Saskatchewan, Alberta, and British Columbia.

The number of female applicants has leveled off in recent years, with correspondingly consistent proportions of women in schools' entering classes. Women made up 56.8% of the 2016–2017 applicant pool, and the success rate for women was slightly higher than that for men. The 2016 entering classes at the 16 Canadian medical schools reporting data about male and female matriculants included 58% women and 42% men. Overall, 22% of applicants received at least one offer of admission.

Expenses and Financial Aid

Tuition and student fees for Canadian and non-Canadian students in the 2017 entering class are provided in Table 14.2 and in individual medical school entries on the Medical School Admission Requirements™ website. Expenses vary from school to school and from student to student. Tuition at several Canadian schools is slightly higher for the first year than for successive years. Some financial aid information is provided in the individual school entries. Eligible Canadian students may apply for a Canadian student loan, or they may apply to the Department of Education in their province for a provincial student loan.

Canadian Medical Schools

ALBERTA

University of Alberta Faculty of Medicine
and Dentistry

University of Calgary Cumming School of Medicine

BRITISH COLUMBIA

University of British Columbia Faculty of Medicine

MANITOBA

University of Manitoba Rady Faculty of Health
Sciences, Max Rady College of Medicine

NEWFOUNDLAND

Memorial University of Newfoundland
Faculty of Medicine

NOVA SCOTIA

Dalhousie University Faculty of Medicine

ONTARIO

McMaster University Michael G. DeGroote
School of Medicine

Northern Ontario School of Medicine

Queen's University Faculty of Health Sciences

University of Ottawa Faculty of Medicine

University of Toronto Faculty of Medicine

The University of Western Ontario–
Schulich School of Medicine & Dentistry

QUEBEC

Faculty of Medicine Université Laval

McGill University Faculty of Medicine

Université de Montréal Faculty of Medicine

Université de Sherbrooke Faculty of Medicine

SASKATCHEWAN

University of Saskatchewan College of Medicine

Worksheets at the end of chapters in this guide are available in fillable PDF format at _aamc.org/msar-resources_.

Questions About Canadian Medical Schools to Ask During Interviews

As you research the Canadian medical schools you're interested in attending, use this worksheet to keep track of questions you think you may ask during your interview. Print or save this page for individual schools and review it the night before your interview or bring it with you. You can find many questions here: *aamc.org/students/download/175218/data/medical_school_interview.pdf*.

Name of Medical School: _____

Type of Interview: _____

Date of Interview: _____

Questions about

1. Curriculum _____
_____
_____

2. Student Involvement _____
_____
_____

3. Special Programs _____
_____
_____

4. Financial Aid _____
_____
_____

5. Facilities _____
_____
_____

6. Academic Evaluations _____
_____
_____

7. Student Support _____
_____
_____

8. Residency Placements _____
_____
_____

9. Other _____
_____

Acronyms

AAMC
Association of American Medical Colleges
aamc.org

AMCAS
American Medical College Application Service®
aamc.org/amcas

CiM
Careers in Medicine®
aamc.org/cim

COA
cost of attendance

EDP
Early Decision Program
students-residents.aamc.org/applying-medical-school/
article/early-decision-program

ERAS
Electronic Residency Application Service®
aamc.org/eras

FAFSA
Free Application for Federal Student Aid
fafsa.ed.gov

FIRST
Financial Information, Resources, Services, and Tools
aamc.org/first

GQ
Graduation Questionnaire

HHMI
Howard Hughes Medical Institute
hhmi.org
hhmi.org/programs/science-education-research-training

HIPAA
Health Insurance Portability and Accountability Act

LCME
Liaison Committee on Medical Education
lcme.org

MCAT
Medical College Admission Test®
aamc.org/mcat

Med-MAR
Medical Minority Applicant Registry
aamc.org/students/minorities

MSAR
Medical School Admission Requirements™
aamc.org/msar

MSQ
Matriculating Student Questionnaire
aamc.org/data/msq

NAAHP
National Association of Advisors for the Health Professions
naahp.org

NBME
National Board of Medical Examiners
nbme.org

NHSC
National Health Service Corps
nhsc.hrsa.gov

NIH
National Institutes of Health
nih.gov
training.nih.gov

NRMP
National Resident Matching Program
nrmp.org

NSLDS
National Student Loan Data System
nslds.ed.gov

SHPEP
Summer Health Professions Education Program
shpep.org

TSF
Tuition and Student Fees Survey
aamc.org/data/tuitionandstudentfees

USMLE
United States Medical Licensing Examination
usmle.org

VSLO
Visiting Student Learning Opportunities™
aamc.org/vslo